TABLE OF CONTENTS

Mommy Muscles

Acknowledgements

While writing *Mommy Muscles*, I've felt so many different emotions: hope, joy, fear, excitement, frustration, fulfillment and pride. For me, this book was a continuation of my journey and a part of who I've become as a result of my healthy lifestyle. But I didn't do it alone.

I want to thank my husband, Greg for being the best editor! And for his ingenious creation of the *Mommy Muscles* front cover. Your tireless efforts helped tremendously, your input and knowledge valuable in so many ways. I'm grateful for your support through this long process and for filling in with household duties while I wrote "one more page."

My son Jake - without you, I would not be a mother and there would be no *Mommy Muscles*. You are my everything! Thank you for your patience and motivation. When I didn't want to write, you encouraged me to keep moving forward and finish the book. Thanks.

My parents, Frank & Patty Iacobelli. Thank you for ALWAYS being there for me and for your constant support through the years. You led by example, raising me to be conscientious, disciplined, caring and helpful. Love you!

My best friend Jackie for patiently listening to me go on and on about my book. Thank you for being my best friend forever. You are the sweetest!

All my friends for your encouragement. When I came up with this crazy idea to write a book, you said, "Go for it!" And for providing me with content – you may recognize snippets of conversations we've had. Don't worry – no names are mentioned.

My gym buddies and fitness friends for hanging with me and working out. Your drive and love of fitness provided me with inspiration to keep going in and out of the gym.

Community High School, my "regular" job for over 17 years. Thanks to my co-workers for listening to me drone on about *Mommy Muscles* for years, (you were a captive audience.) In memory of my friend, Dennis Cohen, who dedicated his life to helping others reach their fullest potential. He touched so many with his driving spirit and he lives forever in my wonderful memories of working for him.

Anthony Greco of *Anthony Greco Photography* for shooting creative fitness photos for me. Your originality and imaginativeness is supreme. You are the official *Mommy Muscles* photographer.

Don't start living tomorrow, tomorrow never arrives.
Start working on your dreams and ambitions today.
- Anonymous

Chapter 1 - All About *Mommy Muscles* - the Book!

Mommy Muscles is for every woman who wants to improve herself and change her life forever. This book will help you achieve a healthy lifestyle by focusing on three factors: working out, eating healthy and keeping a positive outlook. *Mommy Muscles* offers practical advice to help you find your motivation to meet the demands of a busy life while balancing your health and achieving your fitness goals. You'll find workout plans, recipes, and tips for being healthy every day, including on vacation and during the holidays.

The goal of *Mommy Muscles* is to motivate all women, no matter how busy, to take care of themselves. Now is the time to make a positive change and adopt a healthy lifestyle (you'll hear that phrase "healthy lifestyle" over and over again). It is your time to lead a life where you are physically and mentally strong, happy and fulfilled. Don't "wait until Monday" or "after the holidays". There are no rules that say you can't start being healthy on a Tuesday. Make the commitment, stick to it, and you will be forever glad you did.

The first step: set your goals. Maybe you want to lose 15 pounds, run a marathon or just improve your overall health. Second, you have to really want it... and once you make that commitment, you can accomplish your goals regardless of your starting fitness level, how many children you have, or how old you are. With the tools in this book, you'll be able to make a positive change in your life. It is possible to become physically and mentally fit, while being a mom, working outside of the house and managing a household. If I can do it, then you can too - whether you have four kids, no kids, married, divorced or single. I'm sharing my story with you based on my experiences over the years through trial and error. So many women approached me at the gym or at my son's school and asked me questions. I finally decided to write it all down and give birth to *Mommy Muscles*. Think of this book as a mom's group where we're sitting around, chatting about our lives. Or, as a girls night out where we laugh, talk and share our experiences.

A Little Background

Why am I telling you my story? Because my story may also be your story.

I started tap dancing lessons at age three, quickly added jazz and ballet and continued dance until I was seventeen. Dancing kept me fit and I developed good posture and balance at a young age. I never had a weight problem as a child and I was 101 pounds in ninth grade. My gym teacher called my mother to ask if I could possibly be anorexic. Thankfully my mother knew it wasn't an issue. I was definitely eating. Potato chips and dip was my favorite nighttime snack, but I remained thin because of the dancing. I was only 14 years old so I had a fast metabolism and was fortunate enough to eat whatever I wanted and still be skinny.

When I was 16, a new dance instructor was hired at our studio. She lived in New York City and didn't wear the traditional leotard and tights like my other dance teachers. She wore briefs with stockings rolled down over them and a sports bra that revealed her tight abs. I liked the look and I liked her. Her dance choreography was edgy, and her body was tough looking, translation – she had muscles! I saw them and I wanted my own. One day after class I asked her about her regimen and she told me she lifted weights in addition to dancing. This was 1988, the height of aerobics and long before weight training became popular. Lifting weights was something different and I was enthralled. I started doing research by going to the library and book stores, (this was before the internet) and I read everything I could find about weight lifting. At that time, it was often called body shaping for women, and I dove right in. I first started with very light weights, 2.5 lbs., then gradually moved up to 5 lbs. and then 8 lbs. In the early nineties (my college years), ESPN had various exercise shows like *BodyShaping*, *Flex Appeal*, and *Co-ed Training* that focused on weight training. I religiously taped the shows and worked out every day in my bedroom. My boyfriend (now my husband) bought me a home workout bench and I created my own weight lifting routine based on what I had learned through television and books.

My body responded quickly to the weight training routine. By the time I was in my early twenties, I started getting compliments on my arms and stomach. That felt great but I still hated my legs. They weren't long enough or thin enough and I became very self-conscious about the lower half of my body. I was eating what was considered healthy then, although looking back, it was nowhere near as healthy compared to what I eat today. However, it was a different time and we didn't have the knowledge about nutrition that we have now. Everyone thought eating a bagel was a good breakfast! I always got cinnamon raisin without the butter because I wanted to "be good." We now know that a bagel for breakfast isn't a healthy option because they are high in calories and low in nutrients and fiber but we'll talk more about food later.

I continued to enjoy my home workouts in my early thirties and learned even more about healthy eating. Around this time, my husband and I wanted to start our family. I figured I was healthy and would have no problems getting pregnant. Oh boy, was I wrong. To this point, I was able to control my body, working hard to stay in shape and I liked that control. But trying to have a baby was a different story. I could not get pregnant. After a year, we went to a fertility specialist. I had cysts removed and some endometriosis taken care of, but the doctors couldn't find anything else wrong that would cause my infertility. My diagnosis was "Unexplained Infertility" and it was an extremely depressing time. The fertility treatments weren't working. I tried yoga to help relieve my stress and continued with my weight lifting and exercise videos. I thought about my problem all the time, except when I was working out. It became a safe, comforting place for me. Then suddenly, after three years of trying, I got pregnant without medical intervention. It was truly a miracle and we were thrilled!

I was overjoyed about being pregnant, but that wasn't going to be easy either. I was very sick and nauseous. For me, being nauseous is one of the worst feelings in the world and I had it 24 hours a day for close to five months. Ironically, I had to force myself to eat more when I was nauseous, because if I didn't eat, I would get the dry heaves and become very weak. Unfortunately, I could no longer eat the healthy foods I loved, so many of them made me sick. Instead, my diet consisted of potatoes, potato chips, pasta, Italian heroes, and cookies. Just the thought of chicken made me sick. Worst of all, I did not work out at all during the pregnancy. I tried, but I was too sick and too tired. Pregnant Jill was very different from regular Jill. Everything that I did and loved was totally different during those nine months and the result of that was the 65 lbs. I gained. Honestly, it may have even been more. When I saw the numbers on the scale that high, I couldn't even weigh myself the last couple of weeks. It was mentally and physically exhausting.

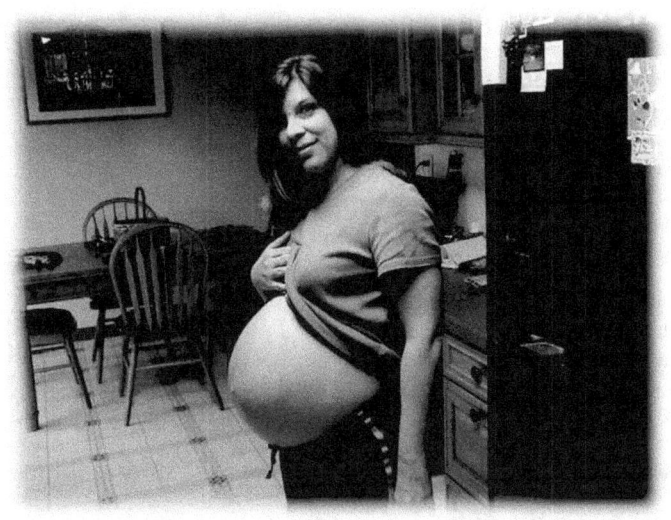

Me with my 65+ lbs. weight gain.
In labor. About 4 am. He finally arrived at 1:01 pm.

After my 8 lb. baby boy was born via emergency C-section, I took a few weeks rest and then made a resolution to lose the weight. It was a challenge that I set up for myself because I didn't want to be like other women I knew who never lost their baby weight. I did it the old fashioned way – I ate less and moved more. I didn't hire a trainer or take diet pills. I was anxious to work out again after having such a long hiatus but found it difficult with a newborn. I was so tired all the time. I'm the type of person that needs a lot of sleep and I don't function well without it. Plus, having a C-section is major surgery and that slowed me down too. As fit as I was before my pregnancy, I had to start all over again since I hadn't worked out for nine months. Eventually, I got my son and me on a schedule. I would exercise when he napped and it worked out perfectly at first. As he got older, it became difficult because his naps were shorter or he wouldn't fall asleep until after I took my shower and got dressed. I tried to get creative with ways to get my workouts in. I would work out in front of him, but at five months, babies don't have long attention spans. I'd have to keep stopping to move him to another activity. We went to a mommy and me yoga class, but he was already walking at nine months so while all the other babies sat and watched their mothers, mine was running away. The sweet yoga instructor ran after him while I perfected my downward dog. I tried using a jogging stroller, but I wasn't a runner at that time and it felt awkward running without being able to swing my arms. I never gave up trying to find different ways to work out. I was committed to getting back in shape and nothing could stop me. I was motivated and determined... but still so tired!

I experienced a steady weight loss and five months after my son was born, I wore a two-piece bathing suit. I felt good, but not great, because I still needed to lose 12-15 more pounds. And those last pounds were the hardest. Eventually, I went a little drastic and cut out carbohydrates but finally lost all my weight plus 5 more pounds. I was thrilled!

My son was going to be turning two and my husband gave me the best present for my 35th birthday – a gym membership. My first reaction: nervousness. I had been working out pretty much all my life but I had never worked out in a gym. Why? Partly because I never felt I needed to since I had my own little gym in my home. I liked working out alone, maybe because I'm an only child or maybe because it was just what I had become accustomed to. The thought of going to a gym was exciting -- but also a little scary. I thought everyone would be looking at me, I thought I might look like an idiot, and I was afraid I wouldn't know how to use the machines. I used to tell my husband that I was gym-phobic but at this point, I needed to make a change. It was becoming too difficult to work out at home with a baby and I wanted to take my fitness to a new level, to challenge myself. It simply was something I couldn't do at home anymore.

Luckily, I live in an area where there are many gyms to choose from and I visited them all. A few things were important to me: a good child care program, low monthly dues with an option to cancel at any time, (in case I hated it), and a general feeling of comfort. You know, sometimes you just get a good or bad vibe from a place. Although I was being practical in my decision, I also listened to my gut feeling. I decided on a coed gym that had a great child care area with wonderful, caring people. I remember the first day I was going to work out, having that butterfly feeling in my stomach. I signed up for the free introduction session and got a quick crash course on the equipment from one of the trainers. Slowly, I got to know the gym and the people that worked out there. Soon, it became familiar and comforting. I learned so much by watching people and talking with them. I wasn't afraid to ask questions. Weight lifting has always been my passion but there weren't many women there lifting heavy weights so I became friendly with a group of guys who were regulars. They took me under their wing and taught me a lot about the machines and different exercises I could do at the gym that I couldn't do at home.

It was interesting that something I had doubts about, belonging to a gym, quickly became something I loved so much. For me, it was a big decision that paid off. It taught me a lesson -- don't be afraid to take that big step out of your comfort zone. Many times I "think" too much. Learn from my experience. Don't let fear stop you...just go for it and you may surprise yourself.

At that point in my life, I was enjoying the gym, working out regularly and eating fairly healthy. I was in my late thirties in pretty good shape, though I started to notice that I'd been slowly gaining some weight. Not a lot, about 8 lbs. but on my small frame, it was enough. I am short, only 5'4", and have short legs so I tend to gain my weight in the butt and legs area. I started to really look at myself and I absolutely hated the way my legs looked. I was so conscious of it that there was an entire summer that I didn't wear shorts, not even for one day. I couldn't believe I gained weight, considering that I was working out regularly and doing my best to stay away from unhealthy foods. I kept trying to lose those 8 lbs. but I wasn't successful. I would lose three, then gain two and it became quite a cycle that I could not break. I wasn't consistent with trying to lose weight and I certainly wasn't happy. To make myself feel better, I would say my motto was to show off the good parts and hide the bad parts. I showed off my muscular arms and fairly toned abs and hid my butt and legs. To most people, I looked fine, but to me, I didn't look good and I didn't feel good. My husband would say, "You are in your late thirties now. You are not as young as you used to be." He was trying to be nice and tell me that he loved me no matter what, but... I really didn't like that response and knew I needed to do something differently.

What I've now learned, is that, as we age, we cannot follow the same workout routine or the same eating plans. So many women tell me they've done everything they can and they just can't lose weight because they have gotten older. That's not true. The reason is because they haven't learned how to change anything about their lifestyle. I am a good example of this. I was working out and eating pretty healthy but still gained weight as I got older. But -- I wasn't going to use age as an excuse and I was going to fight it with everything I had, body, mind and soul.

The first thing I did was to start evaluating my food habits. I was shocked at what I found. I thought I was eating healthy, but I really wasn't. As a matter of fact, I was a little bit out of control. Although I ate well sometimes, I wasn't consistent. At times, I would look for things to eat, even if I wasn't really hungry and I would use the act of eating food as something to do. I was telling myself it was okay because I worked out or that I would only let it happen this one time during the week. I found that I would sometimes stuff myself to the point of feeling uncomfortably full and bloated, looking around the kitchen to see what else I could eat. I would say, "Well I've blown my diet already so I'll just eat whatever tonight and then I'll be real good in the morning." Of course, that one night turns into many more nights. I didn't even realize when I was doing it that this was a very unhealthy habit. Somehow, I had adopted it and to this day, I don't know how or why. Nonetheless, I was doing it and that was definitely a reason I had put on those extra pounds.

Another unhealthy habit I'd formed was to snack at night after dinner. Since I had convinced myself that I had a "sweet tooth," I allowed myself to have something sweet just about every night. This included eating whipped cream, squirted out of the can, or a few spoonfuls of sprinkles. I was consuming too many sweets to satisfy those sugar cravings (more about sugar addiction later). Ugh – looking at it now I know how unhealthy it was. But at the time, I didn't feel like it was really that bad. If we had friends over, I would have dessert with them, usually a small piece of cake and then after they left, I would have another piece of cake. I didn't even sit down and cut a piece, instead I would stand at the counter with a knife and slice tiny pieces, which of course added up to one or even two pieces.

I would blame it on stress, PMS, my husband, and the family barbecues when I should have taken my own responsibility for it. Ultimately, we are all responsible for ourselves. Remember, as we get older, our bodies change and we have to do things differently than when we were younger. It's not fair, but if you're 35 years old, you can't eat like a 25 year old! My self-evaluations told me that not only did I keep the same eating habits I had when I was younger, but I had also developed bad habits of overeating and eating too much sugar. I knew why I gained the weight, now I just needed to change my bad habits into good ones forever. And it was coming at a perfect time in my life.

Turning 40! Turning forty was a big deal for me. It made me stop and evaluate my life in all aspects. I think forty is a good time to re-asses your life and make a positive change. I decided that I was going to do things that were best for my family. I made some changes, cutting out negativity and adding in positivity. My 40th birthday party was one of the best birthdays I ever had because of my wonderful friends that came to celebrate with me. I was, and still am, overwhelmed by their kindness and friendship.

I also decided that I didn't want to be one of those women who said, "Oh well, I'm forty, I can't help it if I have a little belly." I didn't want to start wearing "mom jeans." I was not going to use my age as an excuse. I decided this was the perfect time to get serious about my body and being healthy. I was not quite at the level I really yearned to be, so turning forty became my driving force to step it up and really challenge myself.

At this time P90X was really popular but I didn't want to spend $150 on DVD's. I already belonged to a gym and had a treadmill and elliptical at home. I was thrilled when I found another DVD boxed set called *Supreme 90* at *Bed, Bath and Beyond* and it only cost $15.00. Who knew I'd find my catalyst to extreme fitness at a home goods store! My husband and son bought it as part of my Mother's Day gift. I had mentioned that I wanted it when I saw the advertisement in the store's flyer. I went to the store after work, only to find my husband and son already there buying it for me.

There are ten different DVD's, created with the principles of HIIT (high intensity interval training) and each one focuses on different body parts, such as legs, biceps and back, cardio, etc. I started doing these workouts in addition to my regular gym workouts, where I would do my cardio separate from my weight training. These DVDs incorporate cardio with weights and each movement is done in quick succession so that your heart rate stays elevated, which equals success and sweat. My husband tried the workouts too and we both agreed they were challenging. I thought I was in shape but my endurance was lacking and these DVD's helped me work on that. In addition, these home workouts enabled me to use heavier weights in the gym. I started feeling really good and noticed that my pants were getting big even though I wasn't losing any weight. I know that I shouldn't focus on the scale but during this time, I have to admit that I was a scale watcher. I incorporated running regularly into my routine. I never liked running and in the past, wasn't able to run for very long but I kept pushing myself. I would play a game where I could only run as far as I did the last time and not anything less. Soon, I was doing more and more and worked up to over an hour. Finally, at the age of 40, I could run for 65 minutes without stopping.

My workouts now consisted of running, high intensity interval training in the form of the DVDs and weight training -- a challenging combination that provided tremendous results. I couldn't stop and looked forward to the next workout, each one getting more intense. For the first time, I wasn't afraid of really working out, being out of breath, and pushing out of the comfort zone. And sweating! All at once, I started losing the weight and it came off pretty quickly. I lost eight pounds and dropped two sizes. People started noticing and told me what good shape I was in. I was surprised how many people commented on my muscular arms and told me how tiny I was. My friends asked me how I did it. I was happy to share my story and tell them how I changed my eating and revved up my workouts. I began conducting free boot camp workouts every Sunday morning in the park. I wanted to help others get that "high" that I felt about fitness and being healthy. It wasn't easy but it felt really good! On top of that, we were in the middle of a major house renovation and it wasn't going smoothly. I didn't have a kitchen for nine weeks so it was extremely tough to eat healthy. But I'm proof that it can be done… and you can do it too.

I decided to learn more about fitness and became certified as a Fitness Instructor. I was already unofficially teaching classes but I wanted to do it in an official capacity. I enjoy teaching different classes and I continuously develop different content for my classes that are challenging, innovative, invigorating, and fun. I've taught a variety of classes including Weight Training, Tabata, Interval Training, Kickboxing, Pilates and Core.

Is it hard to be fit at forty? Yes and no! It will be difficult in the beginning but once you are in that zone, it will become easier and part of who you are. Life is difficult and you have to take that difficulty as a challenge and control the things you can. If you stay

17

focused on your goal, you can achieve it. Once you take control of yourself physically, you will feel so much better mentally. It will all come together for you. Believe that you can do anything you set your mind to.

So... that's my story and how *Mommy Muscles* was born. As my body was shrinking, I was growing and developing, working on improving myself and helping others. I absolutely love leading a healthy lifestyle and sharing it with others. I know you want to be healthy too and *Mommy Muscles* can help you with this but you have to be willing to do the work. It won't be easy but it will be worth it. All good things are.

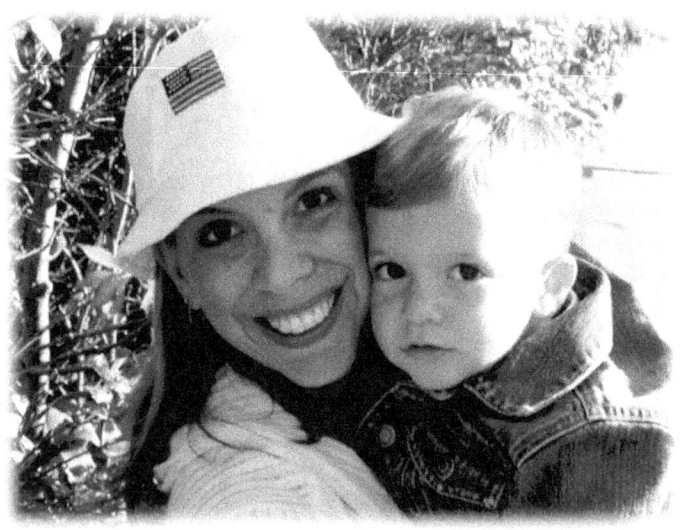

Thanks to this little guy I can proudly carry the Mommy title.

When you find yourself stressed,
ask yourself one question:
Will this matter in 5 years from now?
If yes, then do something about the situation.
If no, then let it go.
- Catherine Pulsifer

Chapter 2 - Mommy Guilt

Don't feel guilty for doing something for yourself. Moms tell me they "feel guilty" working out because they have such a small amount of time with their children and husbands. In today's world, our time is precious between work, school, our children's activities, household chores, errands and other obligations. I ask them, "What does the word guilt mean?" By definition, guilt is "an awareness of having done wrong or committed a crime, accompanied by feelings of shame and regret." Think about that phrase, "having done wrong." Could working out and bettering yourself mentally and physically be wrong? If you took one hour four times a week would your children be any worse off? Being a mother is a hard job and we want to be there all the time and do everything for our children but sometimes, that is not possible.

For example, let's say you have three kids, two have a baseball game on two different fields at the same time and your third child is sick with the stomach flu. What do you do? You probably would stay home with your sick child, have your husband go to one game, and maybe a grandparent go to another. You can't be everywhere at the same time. To top it off, your older son hits a home run and you missed it. Do you feel guilty? Sure you do but it was a situation that was unavoidable and you did the best you could with it. Nonetheless, you feel guilty because "mommy guilt" is something, as mothers, that we deal with every day. We feel guilty because we have other children to take care of, or elderly parents, work obligations, and yes, working out. It's okay to have these feelings but don't use them as an excuse not to exercise. It is important, especially as mothers, to set an example for our children to lead a healthy life. If you want to work out, find a way to do it. Your children will see that it makes you happy and they will understand. What I've learned through the years is, if I take the time to work out, it's okay if I can't get everything done. Family comes first. Usually I'll slack off on my housework. (My mother will cringe when she reads this part). I don't have a cleaning lady, a babysitter or a personal chef. I do the cleaning and cooking myself, but thankfully, my husband helps and my son has his chores as well. I like having a clean house and being organized. I feel a little "off" when the house is messy, but if I don't make my bed one day because I went running before work, I tell myself it's okay. If you're a morning person, you could exercise before the kids get up. But if that's not an option for you, try working out after they go to bed. Either way, it's a chance to spend time on you and get that workout in. And you don't have to feel guilty about not being with your children.

If your children are very young and you're home with them, you could consider childcare at the gym. When my son was a baby, I would bring him to the gym with me and he would play in their childcare room for an hour. He loved it and didn't want to leave. As he got older, he didn't enjoy the playroom as much. I would reason with him and say, "If you go to the gym with mommy, I will take you to the park." He loved that idea and he didn't know that I was going to take him to the park anyway. Children have to learn how to compromise and asking them to stay in the childcare for an hour is not unreasonable. The compromise could be something simple, watching their favorite TV show with them or letting them play in a sprinkler. It becomes a win-win situation and your children will feel important that they can negotiate their reward.

Just as it is important that our children cooperate, it is also important that our families do too. Express to your husband your desire to work out so he understands how important it is to you. Maybe he can get the kids dressed before school in the morning or he can start dinner or put the kids to bed two nights a week. Ask a retired grandparent to help one morning or evening. An older child could set the table, do the dishes or babysit younger children while you do a workout at home. Let your family help you. Every little bit helps to free up time for you.

Get the whole family involved in your healthy lifestyle. Don't cook a meal just for you, cook a healthy meal for the family. Let your kids help with preparing dinner.

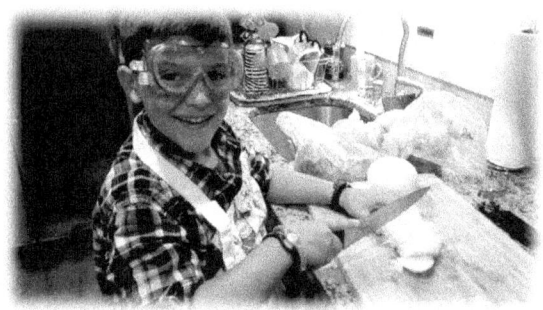

Jake cutting up onions for chili.

Have a family workout night. Kids can take turns being the "instructor" and lead an exercise class. When my son was seven years old, he would help me workout. He acted as my personal trainer and had me do exercises he did in gym class or at football practice. It wasn't easy either! If you engage your children and make them a part of it, then you won't feel that guilt. Once it is a regular part of your life, your family will be used to it. If you make it part of your routine, then the whole family will know that it is part of their lives. Make sure to be consistent. That means, every week, every month, and every season.

Forget about mommy guilt. You shouldn't feel guilty for working out and being healthy. There is a way to have a balance. That equation is different for everyone. Life is busy but there are definitely ways to make it work. Find what works for you and your family and stick to it. Don't use the "guilty excuse" as a reason to not be healthy. Make the time and it will be worth it. Mommies have muscles, not guilt!

Let food be thy medicine, thy medicine shall be thy food.
- Hippocrates

Chapter 3 - Eat Right

What do we tell our children to do? – "Eat your veggies." We want our children to eat well so we cook them healthy meals and try our best to limit sugar. Do you do the same for yourself? The same rules should apply. As much as working out is important to your overall health, your eating habits are even more important. Women ask me all the time how to get flat abs. I tell them it's not about crunches, rather, it's about the food they eat. I get funny looks when I give this answer because I don't think they believe me. But it's true! Healthy eating is 85% (or more) of the equation to keeping you lean and fit. Portion control is a huge factor. Not only do you have to watch the foods you eat, but you have to watch how much you eat.

First, it is important to understand a little bit about calories. The FDA recommends between 1,800 – 2,300 calories a day for women with those numbers varying based on age, height, current weight and daily activities. In order to lose weight, you have to create a deficit. There are approximately 3,500 calories in a pound of stored body fat. If you create a deficit of 3,500, then you will lose one pound. If the deficit is 7,000 calories, then you will lose two pounds. You "create the deficit" or lose the weight through a combination of calories in (reduction of calories) and calories out (increase in physical activity). Another way of looking at it is to reduce your calories by 15-20% below your daily caloric usage.

However, it's not as simple as calories in vs. calories out because not all calories are equal. Foods will have different effects on your body even if they have the same calorie count. For example, you could eat 100 calories in the form of 5 Starburst fruit chews or 13 large steamed shrimp. Realistically, which food would be satisfying? You might get a "high" from eating the candy but it won't fill you up and won't provide any nutritional value. Candy doesn't offer anything of value. Shrimp provides 20 grams of protein, omega-3 fatty acids, vitamin B12 (which helps protect against heart disease) and selenium (which enhances immunity and thyroid function). There are "diets" which count calories and advise you to have 1,500 in a day but it doesn't tell you where to get those calories from. You could easily eat cookies and pretzels all day and still make your goal on these kind of diets. Ideally, you want to eat a variety of different foods that provide nutritional value and energy. Don't get caught up with counting calories. It's good to be aware of them but don't rely on it for weight loss.

The only time I recommend to keep track of daily calories would be at the beginning of your journey. It can give you a baseline to how much you are eating. You may be surprised to discover you eat more than you think throughout the day. You can use a free online program like *FitDay* or *MyFitnessPal* to access these applications on any smartphone, tablet or computer. There is usually an option where you can simply scan the barcode of the food and it will automatically calculate calories, fat, sugars, etc. For this to be effective, you have to record everything, which means all liquids and what I call "quick grab" foods. The quick grabs are the foods that include candy at the office, a few french fries off your children's plates, snacks eaten while the cabinet is still open, and the food you eat while preparing dinner. Once you do this, you will get a clearer picture of exactly what you're eating every day. It takes some work but you won't necessarily have to do it forever. You may find that keeping a food journal can actually help you to eat less, simply because it makes you aware that you are eating.

Another advantage to a food journal is to see how much you are eating at one sitting. If you're eating cereal, pour out your usual serving and measure it. You'll probably have about two cups or more in your bowl. Take a look at the calorie count on the back of the cereal box. You may be eating twice a typical serving size. Depending on the cereal, usually one cup is sufficient. An easy solution is to measure your cereal. Eventually you'll be able to tell just by looking at it. Portion control is a huge factor. Not only do you have to watch the foods you eat, but you have to watch how much you eat.

What Should You Eat?

The *Mommy Muscles* food program is comprised of a clean diet consisting of whole foods that have been minimally processed, lean proteins, vegetables, fruits and whole grains. It maximizes your intake of protein, fiber, and antioxidants and minimizes sugar and white foods. Eating clean will not only help you with your weight but it can reduce your risk of developing diseases such as high blood pressure, high cholesterol and diabetes. In addition, you'll have more energy and look and feel younger.

This program does not tell you what to eat. It tells you *how to eat*. You won't find specific food plans. If I created a food plan with particular foods, and you don't like those foods, then you wouldn't follow it. There are eating suggestions, ideas and information provided for you to make your own healthy choices. Choose the foods that you like based upon the *Mommy Muscles* principles of eating clean, unprocessed foods. The important thing is to find foods you genuinely enjoy eating and that are good for you. This is not a diet, it's a healthy lifestyle of eating clean and balanced foods.

MOMMY MUSCLES FOOD PROGRAM RULES

- EAT APPROXIMATELY EVERY 3 HOURS.
- WATCH YOUR PORTIONS.
- EAT LEAN PROTEINS LIKE CHICKEN AND FISH. (IDEALLY ORGANIC, PASTURE RAISED, GRASS FED.)
- EAT GOOD-FOR-YOU FATS.
- EAT WHOLE GRAINS.
- DRINK WATER THROUGHOUT THE DAY. (ABOUT 8 CUPS.)
- AVOID WHITE FLOUR AND SUGAR.
- AVOID PROCESSED, PACKAGED FOODS.
- AVOID SODA.
- AVOID CALORIE-DENSE FOODS WITH NO NUTRITIONAL VALUE.

Breakfast

Start the day with a healthy breakfast. You've heard it before but it's true. It speeds up your metabolism and give you energy for the day. Mornings are busy for moms. Try preparing your breakfast and your kids' breakfast the night before. Make a big batch of oatmeal at night, or put it in the crock pot and measure it out in the morning. You can even make eggs ahead of time, like a frittata, or eggs in muffin tins and then just microwave them in the morning. If that doesn't work for you, at least have a mental plan so you are not rushing in the morning and making unhealthy choices for convenience.

When my time is limited in the mornings, I'll usually eat a banana with a little peanut butter, Greek yogurt with nuts, decaf coffee and lots of water. When I have more time, I will scramble eggs or make an omelet with veggies and some grated cheese. I also like oatmeal and will make that sometimes. I use steel cut, not the processed ones in the individual pouches.

HEALTHY BREAKFAST OPTIONS:

- OATMEAL - STEEL CUT IS BEST.

- EGGS - SCRAMBLED, OMELETS, HARD BOILED *I USE COOKING SPRAY INSTEAD OF BUTTER TO PREPARE THEM.

- GREEK YOGURT - *BE WATCHFUL AND AVOID YOGURT WITH A LOT OF SUGAR OR ONES THAT ARE HIGH IN CALORIES AND FAT.

You don't want to waste 250 calories on a little bit of yogurt.

- Cottage Cheese - *It's better to get plain and then add your own fruit and some nuts.

- Protein Shake - Almond milk, whey protein, frozen fruit.

- Protein Bar - Pure Protein or Quest are my favorites.

- Fruit - To be added to other breakfast options - don't eat just fruit.

- Homemade Granola - Alone or with Almond milk.

Breakfast Foods to Avoid:

- Bagels - High in calories and no nutritional value.

- Pancakes - Empty calories *Once in a while, splurge on whole wheat pancakes.

- Muffins - Very high in calories and sugar.

- Cereals - Check the calories, sugar and fiber content.

- Granola - High in sugar.

- Sausage and Bacon - High in fat.

Basically, avoid anything "white" - all processed foods like waffles, scones, and donuts. These types of breakfasts are nothing but empty carbohydrate calories with very little protein and fiber. If you eat pancakes for breakfast, you start your day with a high blood sugar level and will have a steep drop just a few hours later. You'll be hungry and crave more of the sugar that you ate for breakfast. Stay away from sugar. I'm not telling you to never have waffles for breakfast but be smart with your choices. If you want to treat yourself to pancakes or waffles, have the whole wheat variety. It is slightly better for you.

However, learn to balance breakfast and all other meals. If you are eating pancakes, especially at a restaurant... don't eat the whole plate. When you have somewhat of an unhealthy choice, practice good portion control. In this way, you haven't done as much damage. Also, make sure that for the rest of the day, you make healthy choices.

Lunch

The typical American lunch usually consists of a sandwich, pizza or burgers. All of which are not exactly healthy. Lunch is often a rushed meal so people tend to grab something that's quick. The problem is that most of these foods don't qualify as "healthy."

Preparing meals ahead of time can help with this. If you are working, pack a lunch. It will save you money too. You could bring leftovers from dinner or prepare lunch such as tuna fish, chicken salad or soup. Make a salad at home. I think salads are fun but they've gotten a bit of a "bad rap." There was a time when people went on restricted diets and all they ate were salads composed of lettuce, tomatoes and typical salad dressings. That's boring and not at all satisfying. It left people hungry. No one would be able to survive on salads alone, which many people tried to do. Then, salads started to become more mainstream. Chain restaurants everywhere offered their version of a Cobb or southwestern salad, but the dressing was so fattening, you'd be better off eating a hamburger. One restaurant offers a Fresh Mex Tostada salad with chicken that contains 1,551 calories, 94 grams of fat, and 2,840 sodium. Wow – that's enough calories for one day, let alone one meal. There are people that think this is a "healthy" alternative.

Today, salads have become creative and customizable. You can add all different kinds of food. Try to see what kind of new salad you can come up with. Pick a theme, like Mexican or Asian and be inventive while making it. There are many different foods you can add. The most important thing to remember is to add a protein to the salad so you stay full longer. Experiment with different types of lettuce, including endive, arugula, romaine, and mesclun. Iceberg doesn't have much taste and there are other greens that are nutritionally better.

Foods to add to salads.

Proteins:

Grilled chicken

Salmon

Tuna

Shrimp

Scallops

Low-Salt Ham

Turkey

Lean Beef

Hard Boiled Eggs

Tofu

Vegetables:

Artichokes

Asparagus

Avocado

Bok Choy

Broccoli

Brussel Sprouts

Cabbage

Carrots

Cauliflower

Celery

Chick peas (Legume -plant protein)

Cucumbers

Edamame

Green Beans

Grilled Eggplant

Hearts of Palm

Kale

Mushrooms

Peas (Legume - plant protein)

Peppers

Radishes

Red Onion

Spaghetti Squash

Spinach

Squash

Sweet Potato

Zucchini

Fruits:

Apples

Grapes

Oranges

Pears

Strawberries

Tangerines

Dried Fruit:

Cranberries

Blueberries

Raisins

Nuts & Seeds:

Almonds

Chia Seeds

Pecans

Pumpkin Seeds

Sesame Seeds

Sunflower Seeds

Soy nuts

Walnuts

Grains

Brown Rice

Corn

Farro

Quinoa

Dairy:

Cheese (low fat)

Dressings:

Balsamic Vinegar & Olive Oil

Fresh squeezed lemon & Olive Oil

Red Wine Vinegar & Olive Oil

Guacamole

Hummus

Salsa

Another thing that makes salads a good choice is that they take a long time to eat! When you eat a sandwich, it's just a few bites and the meal is over. With a salad, there are a lot of forkfuls, which makes it seem like you are eating more. This works especially well when you are out with friends. You can enjoy eating a salad as you talk, instead of noshing on the fried appetizers.

HEALTHY LUNCH OPTIONS

- LEFTOVERS FROM DINNER
- SALAD WITH PROTEIN
- CHICKEN OR VEGGIE BURGER WITH AVOCADO
- TUNA FISH - WITH LEMON
- CHICKEN WITH QUINOA

FOODS TO AVOID FOR LUNCH

- FRIED FOODS
- FAST FOOD
- PIZZA
- HOAGIES/HEROES/SUBS
- GRILLED CHEESE

Every now and then, it's okay to have a treat. Have a slice of pizza or get a hamburger for lunch. These foods are on the "avoid" list because they should only be a "once in a while" thing, not every day or even every week. Don't make a habit of grabbing a burger and fries every Friday.

Dinner

This meal should be more relaxed because you are home with the family. Although with children's activities, dinner also becomes a challenge. Cooking ahead of time or even just planning the meals beforehand, can make a world of difference. Try to enjoy your dinner. Eat slowly. Talk with your family and enjoy the moment of having a dinner, instead of eating quickly and running to the next activity. Sometimes it has to be that way but try to have a few relaxing nights. Be careful not to overeat. People often overeat during this meal. Be mindful of what you are eating and how much you are eating.

HEALTHY DINNER OPTIONS - A PROTEIN AND A VEGETABLE.

- GRILLED CHICKEN AND VEGGIES.
- SALMON AND SAUTÉED SPINACH
- TURKEY MEATLOAF AND A SALAD
- SPAGHETTI SQUASH WITH SHRIMP
- STIR FRYS

FOODS TO AVOID

- FRIED FOODS
- FATTY MEATS

- PROCESSED PRE-MADE MEALS
- FAST FOOD
- PASTA
- WHITE RICE
- HEAVY SAUCES

It's beneficial to eat about every 3 hours. You never want to get "too hungry," where you feel like you could eat everything in front of you. Instead of eating large meals and getting overstuffed, eat small meals and snacks. When you are trying to lose weight, most people restrict their food intake too much and what happens is that your metabolism will respond by slowing down to conserve energy because it doesn't have food coming in. You'll feel sluggish and then you'll overeat at the next meal because you are so hungry. The best thing to do is to keep your intake at an ideal level by eating regularly throughout the day. This will keep your energy up and your blood sugar level. However, it doesn't mean endless snacking or eating just because you feel like it.

Be mindful of your eating habits and be aware of when and how you are eating. By eating a little throughout the day, this will ensure that you won't get too full, too tired, or too cranky. Although it varies based on personal preference, activity for the day, etc.

Here's a snapshot of a typical day of eating small meals:

6:00 am – Water with Bragg's Apple Cider Vinegar, Banana

8:00 am - 6 oz. Low Sugar Greek yogurt, walnuts, coffee

10:30 am - Piece of Fruit, Hard-Boiled Egg

1:00 pm – Salad with Protein or Leftovers from Dinner

3:30 pm – Carrots with Almond Butter

6:00 pm – Chicken or Fish with Veggies

8:30 pm – Fruit or Nuts

"Mommy, can I have a snack?" How many times have you heard that? I have one son and I've heard it a million times. Yes, kids love to snack and when my son was little, I would bring snacks for him in the diaper bag. He would nibble while we were in story time at the library or while I would walk him in the stroller. He enjoyed these snacks and he felt comfortable with them. Think about snacks in a similar way. Enjoy them. Use them to nourish your body and provide you with energy. Always have snacks with you – in the car, at work, and in your bag.

You can be a snacker -- but be a smart snacker. Use snacks as a way to sustain your energy and to provide nutrients to your body throughout the day. It is a great way to fight hunger and to prevent overeating at meals. Just don't snack, "because" and don't mistake healthy snacking as mindless eating. There should be a purpose and reason to your snacking.

Follow these five rules when snacking:

1) **"Why do you want a snack?"**- Are you really hungry or are you just eating because it sounds like fun or you're bored? Sometimes it's just a bad habit, like coming home from work tired and automatically grabbing a snack before dinner. You've probably done it so many times that you don't even know if you are really hungry. You can use the "snack test" to assess if you are truly hungry. Ask yourself, "Could I eat an egg right now?" If you answer, "Yes, I could eat an egg," then you know you're really hungry. But, if the thought of eating an egg doesn't appeal to you, then you probably shouldn't have a snack. Why an egg? It's a food that you probably wouldn't want to eat if you weren't really hungry. You can pick a different food for your "test," maybe tuna fish or broccoli, whatever works for your specific tastes. You don't have to actually eat the food you are using for the test. It's just a tool to gauge your hunger level and your need to actually eat something. Remember, if you ask yourself *why* you want a snack and your answer is something other than hunger (bored, depressed, upset, unsure), then don't snack. Find something else to do.

2) **Control your portions!** - Don't just grab a bag of pretzels, jump into your cozy chair and catch up on your shows. The best way to snack is to portion one serving of what you are

eating into a small bowl, put the rest away, and eat only what you've allotted. And do not go back for more! When you have small children, you don't just give them a box of crackers, instead you portion out a small amount so they don't overeat. Even now, my son's snacks are portioned but he does it himself. He'll put his snack into a bowl and ask me if it's okay before he starts munching.

In addition, try being creative and clever with your portions. The simple trick of cutting up fruits and veggies may help you enjoy snacking more. You can eat a cut apple instead of having it whole. You'll feel like you're eating more if it's in pieces and naturally eat it slower. Or take a cucumber and chop it into tiny pieces, put it into a small bowl so it's overflowing and eat it with a fork. It will make you feel like you are having a substantial snack.

3) **"Are you full?"** - Recognize and monitor when you've eaten enough to be satisfied. If you've portioned a serving of cashews, you don't have to finish what you put into your bowl. If halfway through you're full, stop eating. If you are satisfied and full, there's no need to continue eating. Many times, I'll put three grapes back into the refrigerator. My husband will laugh and say, "You couldn't finish those three grapes?" And I tell him that I'll finish them tomorrow. Know your body and learn what it is telling you. If you are satisfied and full, there's

no need to continue eating. You should be eating to energize your body and supply it with good nutrition -- not just for fun.

4) **Healthy Snacks 100** - Snacks should provide nutrients so stay away from ones with empty calories. If you've determined that you are hungry and you need a snack, then make it a healthy one. Although it sounds like a great idea, 100 calorie packages of cookies and chips are not the best choice. Most times, there's very little in the bag and they lack fiber, protein or healthy fats so you aren't satisfied. You'll end up eating another snack. Many of those packages are processed foods that still contain hydrogenated oils and sugar. Be smart and choose snacks that have nutritional value. Save the cookies for an occasional special treat. A good rule to remember - look in your refrigerator, not your cabinet to choose your snacks. Think fresh and healthy when making your choice.

5) **Prep & Plan** - It's important to have healthy snacks in your home and keep the unhealthy ones out. As soon as you buy your veggies and fruit, wash and prepare them right away to store in containers. They'll be ready when you are hungry or in a hurry. It's also important to have healthy snacks at work, in your car, or even your purse. You never know when you may be out and suddenly your stomach starts grumbling. When you plan your snacks, you'll eat what you bring as opposed to stopping at a store. If you've prepared a healthy

snack and planned ahead, you'll be making the right choices. I tend to over-prepare, but that's a good thing. One time we were going out to dinner with friends and it was already past my dinner time. They live in a rural area where everything is quite a distance away. We all got into the car and started driving. And driving and driving some more. As I watched the beautiful scenery, I could literally hear my stomach growling. I finally asked where the restaurant was. It was still a half hour away! Not only was I was starving but I felt my blood sugar dipping and I really needed to eat something. I grabbed my purse, got out my little plastic baggie and nibbled on some pecans. Aah – I felt so much better and it helped me to not overeat the tortilla chips when we finally got to the restaurant.

HEALTHY SNACK IDEAS:

- FRUIT - GRAPES, BLUEBERRIES, STRAWBERRIES, APPLES, PEARS, CHERRIES, ETC.
- VEGGIES - CARROTS, CELERY, SQUASH, CUCUMBERS, PEPPERS
- YOGURT - GREEK AND BE CAREFUL OF THE SUGAR CONTENT
- LOW FAT COTTAGE CHEESE - ADD FRESH FRUIT
- LOW-FAT CHEESE
- UNSWEETENED APPLESAUCE
- NUTS - ALMONDS, CASHEWS, PISTACHIOS, PECANS, WALNUTS
- AIR-POPPED POPCORN
- EDAMAME - FRESH AND DRIED

Eating Tips & Tricks

One of the most important things to remember when it comes to eating is to never get too full with any meal. You know that feeling, you've overeaten, your stomach is bloated and you feel a little sick. Never get to that point. Eat to the point where you are comfortably satisfied. A good gauge is, "Can you go for a brisk walk right now?" Does your stomach feel distended or is it normal? Learn to stop when you are truly satisfied. In the beginning, you may feel like you want to eat more. It's important to stop before you get that overly full feeling. Eventually, your body will adjust and you will feel very satisfied eating just enough and not more. When you learn how to do this, you will notice that your body will not crave sugar after a meal. You know that little sugar craving you get after you have dinner and want "a little something sweet?" I used to get it all the time, but I don't now. If you eat until you are comfortably full, and not stuffed, that feeling will subside and your body will be satisfied.

The weekend is a time to get things done, relax a little and enjoy. Many times people will "treat" themselves on the weekend.

"Can I have ice cream on the weekends?" one friend asked me.

"Not every weekend," I told her.

"Oh no," she said.

She had been eating ice cream every weekend and wondered why she couldn't lose weight. She was eating pretty healthy during the week, but every weekend she ate ice cream with her family. Of course her weight stayed the same. She felt that since she was "good" all week, she could treat herself on the weekends. So the question is... Can you treat yourself? Of course you can, once in a while. If your family is going out for ice cream, you can have it. But not every time. Grab an extra spoon and share with your family. Take just a few spoonfuls. Tell yourself that today you will have four spoonfuls and then throw that spoon out. You get the taste of the ice cream but are not stuffing yourself. It also teaches your kids a valuable lesson that they don't have to eat the whole thing and it reinforces sharing. Recently, our family went to an Italian ice café and we each got our own ice. I ordered the baby cup even though my husband wanted me to get the medium because it was a better value. I didn't get the medium because it would have been difficult not to eat the whole thing. With the smaller size, I could eat the entire serving without damaging my healthy eating. While we were there, friends of ours came in and all four ordered the large serving. I stared at the size because it looked almost sinful. No one needs to eat that much Italian ice.

Take some time to think about your relationship with food. I'm Italian… need I say more? All my life, every holiday and event has always been about the food. My mother would be having a Memorial Day barbecue and my cousin would call and ask what was on the menu. They'd talk about it for an hour. Once at the barbecue, the food would be barely placed on the table, and my relatives would grab at it. We'd eat about six different desserts (and I'm not exaggerating) and we'd all sit back and say how full we were. After about two hours, people would say, "Hey, I could go for a hot dog." My father would fire up the grill and everyone would eat again. In my twenties, I was part of this food ritual but as I got older, I just couldn't do it. I'd go to bed literally feeling sick and would wake up in the morning and run to the bathroom. It's not always easy for me to be healthy and I certainly wasn't born into it. My parents are from a generation that says, "Just eat it. It's okay, enjoy!" You really can't say no to an Italian mother. So I eat just a little bit. It makes mom happy and it's always a good idea to make mom happy, no matter how old you are. (Read that last sentence to your kids!)

The holidays are always a rough time for staying healthy. There are so many temptations all around. Although I'm a proponent of healthy eating, I love to bake and have been doing so for twenty years. At Christmas time, I absolutely love planning which cookies to bake and usually bake eight or nine different varieties. I give them out to family, friends and neighbors. The only bad thing about baking the cookies is that they are in my house all the time. How do I resist the cookies? I have to set rules for myself just like you set rules for your kids. You certainly wouldn't let your kids eat as many cookies as they wanted, so don't let yourself. Yes, I do eat the cookies and I am a little more lenient with myself during Christmas, but it's important to indulge yourself for a short time. Don't start eating badly in November and continue through March because it was the holidays. Maybe take a week and make a rule that you'll only eat one cookie a day. Or, a rule that you'll only eat two cookies twice a week. The ideal situation, of course, is to not have any cookies but that's not realistic for the vast majority of people. It's also not realistic because you want to enjoy the holidays with your family. I know you don't want to be eating broccoli while everyone else is having homemade lasagna. Have a small piece of lasagna during the holidays. That one piece won't derail you, but continual eating will make the pounds add up. You can indulge "a little" but don't let that indulgence linger for days or even weeks. Take care of yourself, even during the holidays.

Success is the sum of small efforts,
repeated day in and day out.
- Robert Collier

Chapter 4 - How to Cure Sugar Cravings

Do you like to have something sweet after dinner? You know that feeling. You grab two cookies after dinner and tell yourself you'll only have a little something to satisfy your sweet tooth. Then you leave the kitchen but come back to get one of your kids a drink and start thinking about the cookies again. You decide to have two more. That's four cookies already. After the kids are in bed, you sit down to watch TV and again, you think about those cookies. You only eat one, but now you crave chocolate. You grab a few pieces of dark chocolate. Total count is five cookies and three pieces of chocolate in one night. What happened? You ate well all day, then fell apart at night. Now you feel so bad that you figure you might as well eat whatever you want. You forage through the cabinets and eat everything that you've been avoiding. Yikes, that is a very bad situation.

First, your craving for sugar is more than just a craving. It is an addiction, much like an addiction to cocaine, actually. According to a 2012 article on Foxnews.com, Eric Stice, a neuroscientist at the Oregon Research Institute conducted a study and discovered that "sugar is also extremcly addictive - similar to some drugs, like cocaine." Stice took MRI scans of "sugar lovers," people who frequently ate ice cream, drank soda and other sweets. He discovered that "the more sweet foods a person eats, the more he or she builds up a tolerance. The more sugar a person consumes, the less satisfaction that person feels - resulting in eating more and more." If you consume large amounts of sugar, you'll want more sugar and your body literally will crave sugar. It's unhealthy and dangerous.

According to a report by Dr. Sanjay Gupta, (*CBS News 60 Minutes*), an anti-sugar campaign is developing. Dr. Robert Lustig, a California-based endocrinologist believes that the large amounts of sugar consumed by Americans is extremely harmful to our health. He calls sugar "toxic" and says, "It is ultimately killing us." Americans are now consuming 130 pounds of added sugars (including high fructose corn syrup) per person, per year. Much of that sugar consumption is in processed foods. The reason so many Americans are eating large amounts of sugar is because everyone has been trying to reduce fat intake. Since the 1970's, people were warned against eating fats and the government recommended that we lower our fat intake. Unfortunately, the fat was replaced with added sugar, often in the form of high-fructose corn syrup. It tastes good and we love it, becoming almost an "evolutionary Darwinian signal that this is a safe food." If you think sugar is bad for you, just imagine how bad it is for your children. Dr. Robert Lustig says, "The main reason obese children get sick is due to the amount of sugar in their diet." According to his findings, eating large amounts of sugars leads to obesity, type 2 diabetes, hypertension and heart disease.

A five-year study at the University California-Davis has

proved Dr. Lustig's theories true. The study showed that excess consumption of high fructose corn syrup (translation: sugar) increases the risk for heart disease by increasing artery-clogging cholesterol. Kimber Stanhope, a nutritional biologist at the University of Davis, conducted a groundbreaking study. She found that the subjects who consumed high fructose corn syrup, had increased blood levels of LDL, the bad cholesterol, within just two weeks. According to this study, "when a person consumes too much sweet stuff, the liver gets overloaded with fructose and converts some of it into fat. Some of that fat ends up in the bloodstream and helps generate a dangerous kind of cholesterol called small dense LDL. These particles are known to lodge in blood vessels, form plaque and are associated with heart attacks."

If the threat of a heart attack isn't enough to stop you from eating sugar, then what about the threat of cancer? The *60 Minutes* report also interviewed Lewis Cantley, a Harvard professor and the head of the Beth Israel Deaconess Cancer Center, who said that when we eat sugar it causes "a sudden spike in the hormone insulin, which can serve as a catalyst to fuel certain types of cancers." particularly breast and colon cancers. According to Cantley, certain cancers have insulin receptors on their surface and the insulin attaches to the receptors and "signals the tumor to start consuming glucose. Every cell in our body needs glucose to survive. But the trouble is, these cancer cells also use it to grow." So a tumor will get stimulated to absorb the glucose and grow.

According to the American Heart Association's website, many people eat more sugar than they realize and it's important to be careful when choosing foods. In order to see if a food has added sugar, search the list of ingredients not only for sugar and high fructose corn syrup, but also molasses, cane sugar, corn sweetener, raw sugar, syrup, honey, fruit juice concentrates, and words ending in "ose" like maltose or sucrose. It's important to note that each gram of sugar contains four calories. If the food contains 15 grams of sugar, that's 60 calories just from the sugar. The American Heart Association recommends limiting sugar to no more than 100 calories a day, about 6 teaspoons for women, (150 calories for men).

The research I did for this chapter was interesting, informative and a learning experience for me. I had already been limiting sugar for my family but this research made me do a double-take on the foods I give to my son. Just when you think you are doing good... you can always do better. Right before I wrote this chapter, I agreed to make adorable frog cupcakes for my son's second grade class. They looked so cute, but all I could think about was all the sugar the kids were consuming and it literally made me cringe. Cupcakes are such a staple for kids and they really enjoy them. But why do they have to be full of sugar and artificial colors? What about a cupcake *without* the icing? Or a cupcake with a dollop of fresh whipped cream and a blueberry on top? How about using a little bit of peanut or almond butter? I don't think cupcakes will ever stop showing up at birthday parties, but how about reinventing them with a little less sugar?

How do you stop yourself from eating sugar? After reading about the dangers, maybe you're running to your cabinets to purge them of all processed foods with sugar. A great way to avoid sugar is to not have it in your home. If it's not there, you can't eat it. Find other foods to satisfy your sweet tooth. Freeze grapes or banana slices. They are especially sweet when they're frozen. Unsweetened applesauce, sugar-free jello or pudding are all better options.

Another way to stop those sugar cravings -- control your portions. As you get comfortable with your portion sizes, and stop overeating, you'll notice that you won't crave something sweet after dinner. When you overeat, you'll want more sugar. It's natural, because when we overeat, we usually do so with foods like rice, potatoes, pasta and bread - all foods that contain sugar. Your body has built up a sugar tolerance during the meal and you want more. When committing to getting healthy, you should avoid sugar as much as possible. Don't eat sugar or any foods that contain sugar. Be careful of condiments that contain sugar and avoid artificial sweeteners because they aren't good for you either. If you must, use honey which is natural, but really try to do without. Although fruit has sugar, it is allowable because it is all natural and bundled with fiber. Eat a piece of fruit when you want something sweet.

Go cold turkey to retrain your body. Is this hard to do? Yes, this is tough, but not impossible. You don't want your kids to eat a lot of sugar. You should want the same for yourself. You are worth it and you deserve to lead a healthy life. Make a rule that you will not have anything sweet after dinner or any other time of day because you are training your body to stop craving sugar. Don't have any, not even one bite. Believe it or not, it is easier to avoid sugar entirely. While you shouldn't avoid foods or be strict with your limitations, sugar is definitely an exception to this rule. Think of it as a sugar detox to rid your body of toxins. The best way to do this is to eat "clean" and avoid processed foods as much as possible. Eating clean means eating whole, natural foods such as vegetables, fruits, lean meat, fish, healthy fats and complex carbohydrates. These whole foods require your body to work harder during digestion so your metabolism gets a jolt when you eat foods in their natural state. Check labels of the foods you eat and look at the food before you eat it. An easy way to figure out if a food is processed or natural is whether or not the food is perishable. Perishable foods, like peaches, zucchini and oranges are whole, natural foods. Foods like corn chips, pretzels, and potato chips are processed, non-perishable, with a long shelf life.

Do this detox for at least 10 days, and preferably two weeks. You will be so amazed at how much better you'll feel after the detox that you won't crave sugar anymore. Once finished, assess yourself and see how much you really even want sugar. Ideally, you'd never have another morsel of sugar, but that's not realistic. Sugar may come into your life but you'll be able to control yourself by having a small amount. It's important to make rules for yourself so you don't fall back into old habits. You have to decide what works for you and limit how often you have sweets. When you start and continue eating healthy, you won't feel like eating many sweets.

Once you break the sugar cycle and feel you can control your cravings, you can, once in a while, treat yourself with a little something sweet for a special occasion. If you haven't had sugar, when you have that little bite, it will be satisfying. That little piece you have will now taste very sweet and you may be surprised to discover you don't even like it anymore.

Sugar is evil, plain and simple. Not only does it make you gain weight and prevent you from losing weight, but it's physically damaging to your overall health.

I hope reading this has at least made you aware of the dangers of sugar and prompted you to pay more attention to the foods you eat. Don't just grab something sweet. Take a second look, remember what you've read and take a moment to think about it. Make good choices and realize that a bite of sugar may make you feel good for a brief second, but in the long run will damage your body and well-being.

The dictionary is the only place where
success comes before work.
- Mark Twain

Chapter 5 – Eating Tips

When I'm hungry, I need to eat immediately. My stomach growls, I feel weak and I experience an empty feeling in my stomach, signaling that I need food. Eating every few hours helps keep my blood sugar levels stable and prevents me from overeating when I have a meal. I make sure to have healthy food around me all the time so I prepare my food ahead of time. This way, you will always have good food ready that are quick and easy to grab. Here are some prep tips that have worked for me.

Vegetables - When you buy vegetables, cut them up right away. Fresh vegetables go bad quickly so buy them, bring them home and prep them. It's great to snack on or to have when making salads, stir-frys, or soups.

Fruit - Prep fruit as soon as you buy it too. Wash berries, cut melons. Put grapes in plastic baggies so you can easily grab them for a quick snack. If you can't eat all the fruit right away, put some in the freezer to use at a later time for smoothies or just eat them frozen. I love frozen bananas and grapes, in particular.

Chicken - Buy bulk packages of chicken breasts to bake in the oven. Put them in a large pan and season with pepper and garlic powder.

Cook for about an hour. Cut up the cooked chicken into bite-size pieces and put into baggies, some in the refrigerator and some in the freezer. If weather permits, grill the chicken outside or try an indoor grill. Use the chicken, like the vegetables, to put in soups, salads, stir-frys or even as a quick, protein snack. I used to buy pre-packaged sliced chicken that was already seasoned, but it was salty and expensive. Cooking the chicken yourself is less expensive, healthier and really takes little effort.

Bowls & Baggies - Both are great tools to provide instant portion control. Put dried fruit and nuts in little bowls or baggies. This works well because you will only eat what's in the bowl and won't overeat. If you're eating whole wheat crackers and the serving is 20 crackers for 130 calories, count them out into the baggie so you won't overeat.

I admit I'm not a great cook and my family doesn't always like the meals I make. But the one thing I always try to do is make healthy foods. Nothing fried, no heavy sauces or creams and no added sugar or salt. Since I don't love cooking and I don't have a lot of time, I don't spend hours in the kitchen cooking meals. What I like to do, is take some time on a Sunday, (choose the day that works for you), put my favorite music on and make a few different meals for the week. It's not gourmet, but it's healthy, simple meals that I know everyone in my family will like. I make a variety of foods so everyone has something they like. For instance, I love sweet potatoes and squash and bake them in the oven. My husband and son don't like them so I'll also make grilled broccoli and string beans for them. I might make chicken cutlets using oat flour or whole grain rice flour, simple grilled chicken, meatloaf, tuna salad and chicken soup and we'll eat these meals throughout the week. If you have school-aged children, you may have a crazy dinner schedule because of their activities. If you prepare the meals ahead of time, the healthy food will be there and you won't have to stop for fast food on the way to the game.

Our family eats out about once a week. Sometimes I don't feel like cooking or our schedules are busy and it's just easier to go out. Can you still eat healthy when you go out to eat? Yes, you can but plan ahead and make smart food choices. If it's a special occasion, like a birthday or an anniversary, then you might want to treat yourself. If it's a Tuesday night and you're going out for convenience, then there's no reason for treats - it's just a dinner. The reason you need to mentally prepare ahead of time is because when you get to the restaurant, you'll be with your family or friends and will feel tempted to indulge. You might say, "Hey, everyone is having an appetizer, and a drink and dessert. I should too." But you shouldn't. You'll be sorry later. Instead, decide ahead of time what your treat will be. If you are going to a Mexican restaurant and you love the chips and salsa, plan to eat the chips and salsa. This will be your treat. But, you shouldn't order the margarita and a dessert too. You'd end up feeling full and bloated, especially if you've been eating well. Maybe have a taste of the dessert and plan that you will only have three forkfuls of the decadent chocolate cake and two sips of your husband's margarita. If you make a deal with yourself before you go to the restaurant, then you're more likely to stick to it. You could make a deal with your husband or, even better, your kids. They'll love to be in charge and help you with your eating choices. Tell your kids that you will only have one handful of chips. You will put them on your plate and you will not grab any more. You know that if you try to steal a few more chips, your kids will call you out. Making them a part of your healthy lifestyle is a win all around because they will love helping you and it will make them feel important. It will show them how strong and dedicated you are to being healthy, and it will teach them how to be healthy as they grow into adults.

Now that you have mentally prepared before going to the restaurant, it is equally important to physically prepare what you are going to eat ahead of time. If you go to the same restaurants, you'll already know what is on the menu. It becomes a little difficult when you are going to a new restaurant. The best thing to do in this situation is to see if the restaurant has an online menu. This way, you can take your time to choose exactly what you want to eat and figure out the best option for your healthy lifestyle. Many times it's hard to decide what to eat and we sometimes choose an item because it is "our turn" to order. This could lead to a fattening choice. Or, you are so hungry that you pick the menu choice that sounds good, but it's not necessarily the best choice for you. If you plan ahead, you will have picked a healthy choice, something that you like, and you'll have more time to talk and relax at the restaurant. How do you pick a healthy food at a restaurant? There are a couple of things to look for.

Sodium and added fats. Many foods prepared in restaurants are made with tons of salt and butter. The next day after I eat out, my fingers are always bloated from the salt, especially since I don't cook with it or add it to any of the foods I prepare, so I really notice it. Look for low-sodium items or make a special request to have the chef prepare your meal without salt.

Calorie Count - Although I'm not a strict calorie counter, I like to keep a loose count of what I'm eating in a day. I don't want to eat a 2,000 calorie meal for dinner. Do some investigative work and check the calorie count on the menu. You'll be shocked at how many calories some menu choices actually have. We are fortunate that we live in an age where we can easily access this kind of information. Thanks to smartphones, you can look up the calorie count right there at your table. You can easily do a search for "calorie counter" and will find tons of websites that offer this feature. I was shocked to find that some of my favorite salads were very high in calories. For example, at a popular casual chain restaurant, a simple BBQ chopped salad with dressing is a whopping 1,188 calories, 63 grams of fat, and 1,460 mg of sodium. That is a very unhealthy choice. It's just not worth it. At the same restaurant, they offer a Chinese chicken salad that has 707 calories and 23 grams of fat. Still not the ideal, but better than the first choice.

Remember, *Mommy Muscles* is not a "diet." It is a healthy lifestyle and the reality is that you will be going out to dinner. The best way to handle it is to lessen the damage and make the best choices for you. Stay away from the appetizers because there are very few out there that are good for you. Most of them are fried and have no nutritional value. You really don't need them. The same with dessert. Don't eat a whole dessert by yourself and be wise with your choices. Fruit is best, but you can also have some sorbet or sherbet. The chocolate decadent cake featured on the menu is not a good idea. If it's a special occasion and you are having dessert, make it just a few bites.

What's a good choice for a meal? Here are some rules to follow.

Good Choices:

- Dishes that are grilled, baked, steamed and broiled
- Order protein, chicken, fish, lean beef or pork
- Salad dressing on the side. Order vinegar, lemon and olive oil or a "light dressing"
- Water or seltzer to drink
- Marinara sauce or fresh tomatoes
- Veggies (without butter or sauces)

Avoid:

- Fried or sautéed items
- Creamy salad dressings, like Ranch, Blue Cheese or French
- Soda, sweetened iced tea, juices
- Alfredo, cream sauces
- Bread and butter
- Sour cream, cheese

You have to find what works for you based on the foods you enjoy. It also depends what stage you are in: Are you trying to lose weight? Are you maintaining? What was your eating like during the week? What is your schedule like for next week?

When I go out to eat, I order a protein, like chicken, beef or fish and a vegetable. I don't order a pasta dish and if I'm served rice or potatoes, I eat very little of them. I rarely eat white potatoes, instead opting for sweet potatoes and I prefer quinoa over rice. I'll occasionally have a taste of an appetizer or dessert but I don't order my own. My drink of choice is always seltzer with lemon or lime.

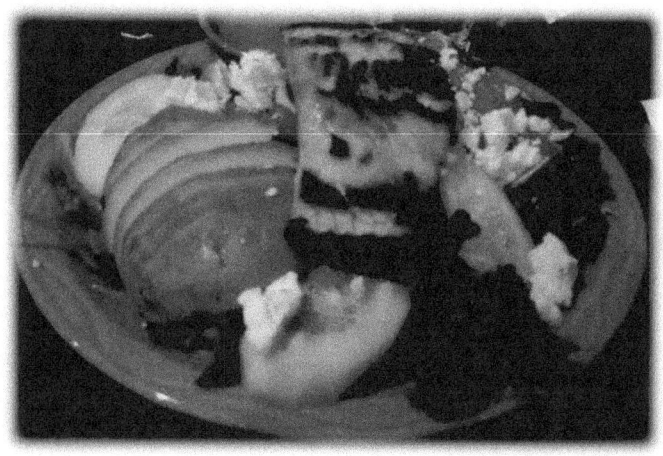

Salmon with salad – lettuce, avocado cucumbers, feta cheese

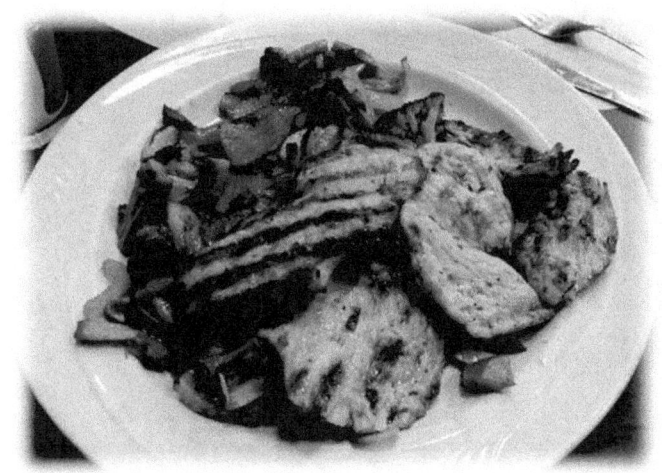

Grilled chicken & grilled veggies from our local pizza place

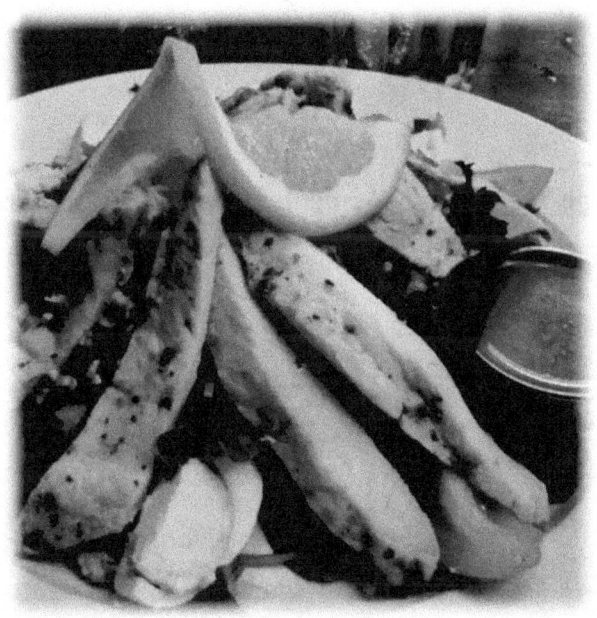

Grilled chicken salad – from a pub in NYC

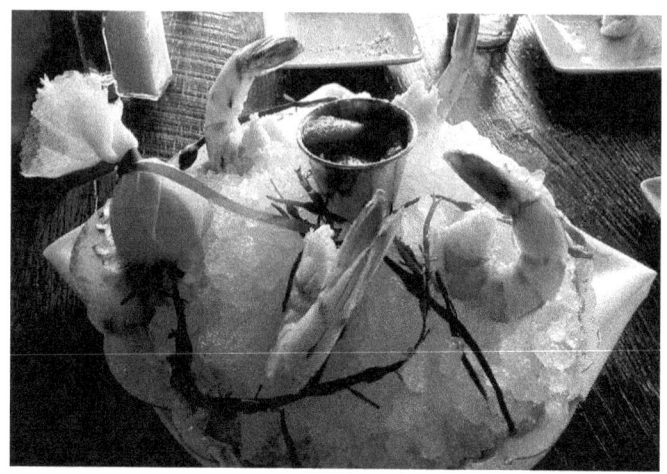

Healthy appetizer – shrimp cocktail

Remember you are eating for your health, not just to lose weight. You should choose foods that are low in saturated fats, trans fats and cholesterol to promote heart health.

The <u>American Heart Association</u> offers the following tips when ordering your meal:

- *Avoid ordering before-the-meal "extras" like cocktails, appetizers, bread and butter because these are often sources of extra fat, sodium and calories.*

- *Ask for butter, cream cheese, salad dressings, sauces and gravies to be served on the side, so you can control the quantity you consume. Instead of fried oysters, or fried fish or chicken, choose boiled spiced shrimp, or baked, boiled or grilled fish or chicken. Steer clear of high-sodium foods -*

including any food that's served pickled, in cocktail sauce, smoked, in broth or au jus, or in soy or teriyaki sauce. Avoid dishes with lots of cheese, sour cream and mayonnaise.

- *Be selective at salad bars. Choose fresh greens, raw vegetables, fresh fruits, garbanzo beans and reduced-fat, low-fat, light or fat-free dressings. Avoid cheeses, marinated salads, pasta salads and fruit salads with whipped cream.*

- *Choose desserts carefully. Fresh fruit, fruit ice, sherbet, gelatin and angel food cake are good alternatives to more traditional fat- and cream-laden desserts. Use fat-free or 1% milk in coffee instead of cream or half-and-half.*

- *Don't be hesitant to ask your server how particular foods are prepared or what ingredients they contain.*

- *Ask what kinds of oils foods are prepared with or cooked in. The most desirable oils are monounsaturated oils (olive oil, canola oil and peanut oil) and polyunsaturated oils (soybean oil, corn oil, safflower oil and sunflower oil).*

- *Ask whether the restaurant can prepare your food to order - for example, by leaving off or going very light on dressings, butter, cheese or other high-fat items. Ask the chef to prepare the food with very little butter or oil or none at all.*

- *Ask if smaller portions are available or whether you can share entrees with a companion. If smaller portions aren't available, ask for a to-go box when you order and place half the entrée in the box to eat later.*

- *Make healthy substitutions whenever possible. For example, if a dish comes with french fries or onion rings, ask whether you can get a baked potato with vegetables, and light sour cream. Instead of mayonnaise-laden coleslaw, ask if you can get a small salad, fruit or vegetables instead. Although some substitutions may cost a little extra, the health benefits are well worth it.*

You've planned ahead and ordered a healthy meal (or at least close to it) at a restaurant. Once your food arrives, be diligent when it's in front of you. Simply, DO NOT EAT THE WHOLE THING! You will be tempted and you will want to eat everything, but you shouldn't. The portion sizes in restaurants have dramatically increased. Eating a larger portion, may make you feel bloated, stuffed, possibly a little sick, and probably a little guilty. How can you stop yourself from eating the whole thing? Once again, you can enlist the help of your kids, your husband and your friends to police you. Divide your food and decide before you even start eating, how much you will eat and stick to that plan!

Another way to control your portions in a restaurant is to immediately ask the waiter to bring you a container. When you are sitting in the restaurant, you have to tell yourself that you will not eat the whole dish right now. There is always an option to save it and enjoy it again at another time. Put some of your food in right away and close the lid. You are making your meal last and you can look forward to eating it for leftovers. By the way, I LOVE leftovers for several reasons: One - I don't have to cook and I get a break from not only cooking but also cleaning up. Leftovers are easy. Just pop them into the microwave and voila, you have a great meal. Two - It gives me a chance to eat something I really like again. It's a reward to myself for not eating the whole thing the first time. Often, I eat it for lunch the next day and enjoy it as much as the first time. If you don't like leftovers, please reconsider. Eating leftovers fits with a healthy lifestyle.

RULES FOR EATING OUT

- MENTALLY PREPARE AHEAD
- HAVE AN IDEA OF WHAT YOU WILL ORDER
- CHECK THE CALORIE COUNT OF THE FOOD YOU ARE ORDERING
- MAKE SMART CHOICES
- ENLIST THE HELP OF YOUR FAMILY TO KEEP YOU ON TRACK
- BRING HOME LEFTOVERS

On Vacation

There is nothing better than planning a great vacation for your family. You plan the hotel, the activities, and the restaurants. Food is a part of vacation and often a time when people go totally off their diets. I know, I've done it in the past. I call it a "food vacation" because you say to yourself, "I'm going to eat whatever I want. When I get back, I'll eat well again." The problem is you never really get on track when you get back home. The "food vacation" seems to linger longer than your week vacation. One explanation is that sugar is toxic and addicting. You get so used to the sugar, that your body is craving it and you have trouble stopping long after you've settled back at home. Or, you are stressed because you're back at work, or depressed that your vacation is over and you are back to your normal life that you eat to fill that void. Either way, it always seems to last way longer than it should. Turn your "food vacation" into a "mini get-away." Yes, you can treat yourself on vacation but no, you cannot go totally crazy.

The other problem with eating everything you want on vacation is that in just one week, you will probably gain a few pounds. I know that for me, in the past, I've gained as much as four pounds on a one-week vacation. Guess how long it took me to lose those four pounds when I got home? A lot longer than a week. It took about three weeks. That really doesn't seem fair but it's true. One week of eating crazy takes about three weeks to lose. I finally realized that it just wasn't worth it. Absolutely enjoy your vacation but don't make the entire trip about food. Get excited for other fun activities or relaxing moments. Set a goal to stay the same weight. If you can do that, then you've accomplished something big. And, I've even had vacations where I lost weight. It is possible!

Follow these rules so you don't gain weight on vacation:

The first rule: Don't go absolutely crazy and eat whatever you want whenever you want. It's just not good for you. If you've been working hard and losing weight, you don't want to step back into old habits. It's the same rule as an alcoholic who can't have just one drink. You shouldn't have even one gorge or pig out meal but you can break the rules a little and indulge in foods you really enjoy. Have a piece of pizza or an ice cream cone, but don't have two pieces of pizza and a large ice cream cone. Remember your portion control. If you are going out to dinner, (mostly every night on vacation), follow the same rules you follow at home when you go to a restaurant. Don't lose control. Stay in the healthy zone. If you do, you can still enjoy occasional vacation treats, but you won't ruin your healthy lifestyle in one week. Remember who you are and what you've become. You've worked too hard to ruin it on a vacation. Indulge a little with some foods that you normally don't eat -- but keep yourself balanced and healthy.

The second rule: Continue to eat breakfast, lunch, dinner and snacks. I know schedules are different on vacation, but stick with your food schedule as much as you can. You don't have the everyday stress of your life, so take some time to concentrate on your food habits. Whether you're on a sightseeing or a beach vacation, prepare and plan ahead so you always have food around. Pack snacks and plan your meals. Our family goes on a lot of beach vacations, so I always do a quick run to the store on the first day to pick up healthy foods.

When we're hungry, we snack on fresh blueberries, grapes and watermelon, hard boiled eggs and low fat cheese sticks. I'll also buy some whole wheat pretzels, rice cakes and peanut butter.

Don't skip meals. People often decide to skip lunch because they are going out to a nice restaurant for dinner and they are "saving" calories. Not the right way to think. If you don't eat lunch, you'll be extra hungry for dinner and you'll overeat. You never want to be starving before a meal -- just hungry. Skipping meals only makes you eat more at the next meal. Continue with your three meals and snacks throughout the day to keep your blood sugar levels even and your hunger pangs in check.

The third rule: Pick and choose. Have you ever told your kids to pick and choose how to spend their money? Maybe you've been on vacation and you tell them they can only go on five rides so they need to "pick and choose" which ones. Or you tell them to "pick and choose" which souvenir to buy at the gift shop. They have to make smart choices. Do the same thing with your food choices. Pick and choose which treats you are going to have. When I vacation at the Jersey shore, once a year, there are certain foods that I eat: pizza, french fries and frozen custard. Over a week, my family may want pizza twice. I choose to have pizza one of the nights and I only eat one slice. I still get to enjoy the pizza, but I don't overindulge. The same is true with the frozen custard. I might eat it twice, always getting the smallest size, and sometimes even asking for a "baby cup." Other times, I don't order my own but I'll take a spoon and share with my family. If you are eating really healthy, you'll be satisfied with just a few bites. If you do order your own, try not to eat the whole thing. This is difficult, but you'll feel better in the end. Remember, you don't want to feel so full that your stomach is bloated and you get that stuffed feeling, especially with desserts. It's after a meal so it's not a hunger issue at this point, it's more of a pleasure principle. You are already satisfied by your meal so the dessert is just a treat. Mentally, go beyond what you are feeling at that moment. Think about how you'll feel the next morning when you wake up and put on your bathing suit. If you've made smart choices, you will be proud of yourself the next morning. There are consequences to all our actions. Good actions lead to good consequences that will benefit you.

The last rule: Be a leader, not a follower. You want your kids to lead and not follow the wrong crowd, right? Well, this is the same thing. On our last vacation, my husband and son were eating bacon, egg and cheese sandwiches for breakfast while I had hard boiled eggs and yogurt. I really didn't mind. I knew I was keeping my body healthy and that I wouldn't gain weight on the vacation. I sometimes took a bite of the sandwich and it was good, but not good enough for me to eat the whole thing. I just kept thinking about how I wanted to look and feel.

If you are vacationing with a group of people and everyone is eating badly at every meal, that doesn't mean that you should do what they're doing. Don't be afraid to do something different. If everyone is getting dessert, you don't have to. Sometimes I split it with my husband and sometimes I just get a cup of coffee. I don't let what other people are doing influence me. I only get the dessert if I really want it, if I'm not too full, and if I haven't had a dessert in a while. Who knows, you may inspire other people in your group to eat healthier too! Don't blindly follow the crowd, be mindful of your goals and what is best for you. In the end, you will be happy and healthy.

RULES FOR VACATION:

- DON'T GO ABSOLUTELY CRAZY.
- KEEP YOUR SCHEDULE - BREAKFAST, LUNCH, DINNER, SNACKS.
- USE THE "PICK AND CHOOSE" RULE.
- BE A LEADER... NOT A FOLLOWER.

The Grocery Store

I hate to sound like a stereotypical woman but, I do love shopping, perusing different stores at the mall to add more clothes to my wardrobe. Grocery shopping, however, is a whole different story. I've never met anyone who said it was fun. Some people have said they don't mind it, but never that they loved it. Yet, it is a necessity, especially for moms. I have a family of three, so I don't have to go too often. Some of my friends are a family of five and they always seem to be running to the store. It's one of those chores that we have to do. It's an important chore because whatever we bring into the house, our family will eat.

If you want to eat healthy, it starts at the grocery store. Make smart choices there and it will be easier for you when you are at home. DON'T BUY JUNK FOOD. If you don't buy it, you won't eat it.

When you are at the store, the food looks good. You might tell yourself that you'll buy the vanilla caramel cupcakes but you'll only eat one and save the rest for your kids and their friends. But the temptation to eat another one will be there in your home. If you don't buy them, then you won't have to worry about eating one or two or five. Eliminate the temptation. Your kids shouldn't be eating it either.

Can you buy treats at the store? Yes, but not every time and be cognizant of the types of treats you buy. I'd rather have a slice of homemade cake than a piece of packaged, processed cake. Ideally, your house should be 100% junk free -- but that is 100% unrealistic. Being extreme only will lead you to seek it out and splurge uncontrollably one day. When you have kids and their friends are over, they usually want snacks. A healthy option would be to feed them carrot sticks and celery but that's not a viable option all the time. Would the kids stopping visiting your house? Maybe. You could put some peanut butter on the celery or make a dip for the carrots. And sometimes, it's okay to serve a special treat. Just be selective with those treats. Pick the *best* option. Take a look at the chart below:

	Calories	Fat	Sugar
Small brownie	170	6.85 grams	15.38 grams
Sugar cookie	43	1.94 grams	2.4 grams
Animal cracker	11	.34 grams	.35 grams

You can see the big difference in the nutritional breakdown of these three snacks. Make a smart choice. A cookie isn't the perfect snack, but if you or your family must have a cookie, choose one that is a little better for you.

Grocery shopping for healthy foods is difficult because it takes time to read the labels. Once you get used to buying healthier choices, your shopping will get easier because you'll know what you want to buy. In the beginning, as you adjust to your new healthy lifestyle, it will take some time to shop. Use the "pick and choose" method when going to the store. Take a few extra minutes to read the nutritional value on the package and make smart choices for you and your family.

Always make a list before you go food shopping. I'm sure you've heard this tip before, but it works. It keeps you focused on the items you're at the store to buy instead of being distracted by the sour cream and onion potato chips. Try using a free application like Evernote that you can download to your phone to keep a food shopping list always at your fingertips. If you stop at the store unexpectedly, you'll have it. I used to keep a list on a scrap of paper.

Of course, I would lose the paper or leave it at home, not having it with me when I actually went to the store. I always have my phone and can continue adding items to the list, especially when in the kitchen. Plus it's handy because you can save items that you buy frequently. Every week, I buy carrots, celery, yogurt, and bananas so they are staples on my list. It's really convenient and a great way to stay organized.

The other advice you've probably heard a hundred times, but I will say it again, is to NEVER go to the grocery store hungry. It's common sense because you'll want to buy everything, regardless of the healthy factor. You'll get home and eat everything, which will be followed by guilty feelings. Ugh, it's a vicious cycle. Stop before it continues. Even though most of the food I buy is healthy, I notice that if I do go grocery shopping when I'm hungry, I'll even overbuy healthy food. I'll buy extra fruit, more avocados than I could ever eat and tons of pistachios. I'm just so hungry and I get excited seeing all the food. Plus, if I go hungry, I have less patience to read labels and find the right choices.

Lastly, go food shopping when the store is not crowded. How many times have you been to the grocery store when it is packed with people and you race through, grabbing food quickly so you can just get out of there? I don't mind food shopping but I hate it when the store is crowded. It can be difficult to shop with people all around, trying to squeeze your cart through the aisles. This can lead to frustration and you may not take the time to choose healthy food. It takes time to read the labels, checking the calories, fat, sodium and sugar contents. As it is, you are probably running to the store in-between dropping your kids at baseball practice. Or you're dragging your toddler with you and hoping you can get through your list before they throw a fit about getting out of the cart. Those are things you have to work around, so schedule a time when you can shop in a less crowded environment. Sometimes early in the morning is quiet or later at night. I know it can be a chore but try to think of food shopping as a pathway to your healthy lifestyle.

RULES FOR GROCERY SHOPPING:

- DON'T BUY JUNK.
- MAKE A LIST AND STICK TO IT.
- NEVER GO TO THE STORE HUNGRY.
- TRY TO SHOP WHEN THE STORE IS LESS CROWDED.

Good Foods:

There are so many foods out there that are good for you. Think of eating as a way to nourish your body. Sometimes women tell me that they know they should eat healthy, and they think they are. In actuality, they aren't. One woman told me she cut all carbohydrates completely. She's setting herself up to fail, because she'll eventually have to eat carbohydrates and she'll end up gorging on them. Carbs are the primary food for energy. There's nothing wrong with eating 'good for you carbs' like oatmeal, brown rice and fruit. The only danger is eating too much of them and eating them at the wrong times. In addition, restricting one food group from your diet is never a good idea because it can also cause nutritional deficiencies. Brown rice and oatmeal are high in fiber and rich in B vitamins like folic acid.

Another dieting mistake: thinking all fat is bad for you. The bad fats, like saturated and trans fats, will make you gain weight and clog your arteries. However, there are good fats, like those in avocado, olive oil, and nuts. We need to have the good fat in our diet. These fats, like monounsaturated, polyunsaturated and omega 3 fatty acids, are beneficial to our diets. Research shows that these good fats fight fatigue and sustain your mental capabilities. Remember, products labeled "fat free" are typically processed and have added sugars. They're not good for you. Choose the healthy fats for a healthy lifestyle.

Eat foods that are healthy but find foods you like. Spinach is good for you, but if you hate it, don't eat it. Experiment to find foods you enjoy eating. Let eating be a pleasant experience. Too often, women use that word "diet" and tell me they hate it because they don't like to eat yogurt. I say, "Don't eat yogurt." It shouldn't be an unpleasant experience -- it's your new lifestyle. There are many foods that are good for you Give them a try and see which ones you like.

It's a mistake to go on a strict "diet." The problem with being overly strict is that you will never stick to the plan. You'll stay on that kind of plan for one or two weeks and then give it up. It's not realistic and it's not real life.

The way to lose the weight and keep it off is to learn how to balance your life, with exercise and proper eating. Make healthy, clean eating part of your everyday life. The most important thing to ask yourself when deciding what to eat is, "Is this food natural, or is it processed?" In the simplest terms, eat lean meats, vegetables, whole grains, fruits, and some healthy fats. Stay far away from sugar, packaged foods, and white carbohydrates. And, watch your portion sizes! That's really all there is to it. You've read all about it. You have the information. Now is the time to get serious and use your new-found knowledge to make a change in your life. Be who you always wanted to be.

Can I have a drink?

I want to spend a little time talking about drinks because it's also an important aspect of leading a healthy lifestyle. It's very simple – drink water and lots of it. Carry it around so you always have it with you. If you have little ones, you probably have a sippy cup nearby right? Do the same for yourself. I don't leave the house without my phone or my water bottle. Buy a reusable one and keep filling it up all day.

Drinking water is vital to maintaining a healthy metabolism and for your overall health. It assists with digestion by aiding in digesting soluble fiber, which can help you lose weight. It enables your body to excrete waste through sweat, and by going to the bathroom (yes, both #1 and #2). Water regulates body temperature, transports nutrients and oxygen into cells, protects our vital organs while helping them to absorb nutrients, cushions the spinal cord and lubricates joints, regulates body temperature, and detoxifies. Wow! Isn't it amazing that something so simple, something we see and use every day, can do all of those wonderful things for us? Remember, approximately ⅔ of our body consists of water so stay hydrated at all times. A good rule (I know this is going to sound a little funny) but if your urine is clear, then you are hydrated. If it's yellow, then you need to drink more.

If you don't like water, try adding pieces of lemon, lime or orange. It gives it a little flavor and once you start drinking water regularly, you'll start to enjoy it. I remember as a teenager thinking water was so "blah" but as an adult, I absolutely love it. I felt the same way about seltzer but now, this is my go-to drink when out to dinner.

A great way to get fluids and keep your body healthy is to mix 8 ounces of water with 1-2 teaspoons of Bragg's Apple Cider Vinegar, (ACV). It's raw, organic, unpasteurized apple cider vinegar. You will notice some sediment floating on the bottom. This is called "the mother" and it is the most important part because it contains raw enzymes and gut-friendly bacteria that promotes healing. Just shake the bottle before using it. Do not drink it alone because it's strong and could damage tooth enamel. When mixed with water, it's fine. I drink it first thing every morning and have found it to be a great start to the day. It has helped with some of my stomach issues. I also like to have it after I exercise, especially after a long run. The taste is a bit "odd" but after a while, you may get used to it. Add lemon or even a little bit of honey to "soften" the taste. Give it a try.

BENEFITS OF BRAGG'S APPLE CIDER VINEGAR:

- RICH IN ENZYMES & POTASSIUM
- SUPPORT A HEALTHY IMMUNE SYSTEM
- HELPS CONTROL WEIGHT
- PROMOTES DIGESTION (REDUCES GAS AND BLOATING)
- PROMOTES ALKALINITY IN THE BODY
- HELPS SOOTHE DRY THROATS
- HELPS REMOVE BODY SLUDGE TOXINS
- HELPS MAINTAIN HEALTHY SKIN

Another great tip - drink warm water with lemon in the morning. It's soothing and satisfying, especially in the colder months.

Benefits include:

- Boosts your immune system because lemons are high in vitamin C and potassium.

- Balances your pH by reducing the body's overall acidity. Even though lemons are acidic, they do not create acidity in the body; instead they are alkaline inside our bodies.

- Aids digestion by helping the liver produce bile, which is required for digestion. The warm water stimulates the gastrointestinal tract and helps lubricate during peristalsis - waves of muscle contractions within the intestinal walls that helps contents move through the digestive tract.

- Acts as a natural diuretic. Lemons help increase the rate of urination in the body. It helps to flush out unwanted materials and helps purify the body because toxins are released faster, keeping your urinary tract healthy.

- Clears skin. The vitamin C helps to decrease wrinkles and other blemishes. In addition, the lemon water rids toxins from the blood which keeps skin clear and healthy.

- Helps with weight loss. Lemons are high in pectin fiber which helps control cravings.

- Beneficial for respiratory infections. Loosens phlegm and rids the body of toxins.

Once in a while, in the summer, I'll make sun tea. I use decaffeinated green tea bags, and put them in a pitcher full of water. Just leave it out in the sun and you'll have fresh home-brewed tea. Add a touch of lemon and honey but no sugar.

Juices contain a lot of sugar. An occasional small glass of orange juice, especially freshly squeezed, is fine. But be careful consuming large amounts of juice -- and definitely keep it away from your kids. Juicing has become the latest rage. I do juice once in a while, mixing two vegetables with one fruit so it's not full of sugar. I'll juice carrots, celery and an apple. Or cucumber, kale and a pear. It has to taste good. Don't drink it, "just because" you've heard it's good for you. Try different combinations and stick with the ones you like.

Caffeine

I don't do caffeine. Yes, you read that right. Whenever I tell people that, they look at me as if I said I don't breathe air. I used to drink caffeinated coffee and tea when I was younger. Like so many, I loved it but around my early thirties, I noticed the caffeine started bothering me. If I drank coffee on an empty stomach, I would feel a little dizzy and shaky, so I made sure to only have it after a meal. But slowly, even on a full stomach, I noticed that I just wasn't feeling right after drinking it. In addition to that shaky feeling, I started getting heart palpitations. This was how I found out I had Mitral Valve Prolapse. At first I just cut down on the caffeine, but soon after this, I finally got pregnant and figured it was the perfect time to cut caffeine completely. I still love coffee but I always order decaf and I don't notice the difference. It has been over ten years that I'm caffeine free. I don't miss it!

Wine or Whine?

You're probably waiting for me to talk about alcoholic drinks, right? I know, sometimes you feel like you want to have a "drink" and you are wondering if you can have alcohol while you're living the healthy lifestyle. The answer is yes and no. Yes, you can have a drink every now and again. No, you can't have it on a regular basis. Alcohol is high in calories and contains lots of sugar. It has 7 calories per gram, making it the second-most calorie-dense macronutrient. (That's just below pure fat, which has 9 calories per gram).

It's important to understand how alcohol is processed in your body. First, your body wants to process alcohol before anything else, including food. Pamela M. Peeke, MD, author of *The Hunger Fix* says, "Drinking presses 'pause' on your metabolism, shoves away the other calories, and says, 'Break me down first!'" The result is that whatever you recently ate gets stored as fat. What's worse: "Research has uncovered that alcohol especially decreases fat burn in the belly," Dr. Peeke adds. "That's why you never hear about 'beer hips,' you hear about a 'beer belly.'" Alcohol definitely bloats you. Have you ever noticed how heavy drinkers have bloated bellies and faces?

Another concern when going out and drinking alcohol is that the high sugar content in drinks will make you hungry. Remember our earlier discussion on sugar? Your body will crave food, probably something salty or sweet -- most likely you won't be craving carrots with hummus. Drinking alcohol lowers your inhibitions and therefore leads to bad food choices. If you're at a bar, usually the only offering is greasy and fried, "bar food."

Everyone loves a daiquiri or a margarita because they taste good but some of these mixes have as much as 35 grams of sugar (equivalent to 7 teaspoons of sugar) and over 500 calories per drink. Not a good choice. A regular beer is about 153 calories and light beer is 103 for just one beer. A 1.5-ounce jigger of vodka has almost 100 calories and a 5 oz. glass of red wine is 125 calories. You can see how quickly the calories add up when drinking alcohol. Alcoholic drinks can be very fattening and, most times, people don't even realize how many calories they're drinking. If you are doing well eating healthy, don't negate that effort with alcoholic beverages.

It isn't realistic to say never have a drink. But if you are going to drink occasionally, be smart about it.

Rules to follow:

- Know your portion sizes. A red wine glass usually holds 12-14 oz.

- Know your limits - have one or two drinks.

- Be smart. Alcohol dehydrates you, so be sure to drink lots of water, preferably a glass of water for every drink you've had. In the morning, drink water first thing.

- Be sure to eat before you drink. Have some protein, fiber and a healthy fat. According to Karlene Karst, RD author of The Full-Fat Solution. Eating will "stabilize your blood-sugar levels without slowing down your metabolism. Karst recommends Greek yogurt with berries, almond or hemp butter with an apple, or a protein shake. An added benefit of grabbing a bite beforehand, she says, is that a Pinot or appletini will be absorbed more slowly into the bloodstream, minimizing its diet-damaging effects."

- Treat alcohol like you would dessert; once in a while is okay but don't do it every Friday and Saturday night.

- *Be careful, be selective and be safe when it comes to drinking alcohol.*

One cannot think well, love well,
sleep well, if one has not dined well.
-Virginia Woolf

Chapter 6 – Recipes and Food Ideas

Here are "Recipes" and "Food Ideas." I cook simple healthy dishes that everyone in my family will enjoy. Not always an easy task. I don't cook with butter, opting for olive or coconut oil instead and I never add salt. Don't fry foods and stay away from packaged pre-made mixes. I usually make enough so there's leftovers.

These recipes are categorized for easy reference. However, be sure to have a complete, balanced meal. Don't eat too much of one food group. Always include a protein with every meal. A salad can be a great option but if there isn't any protein in it, it won't sustain your hunger for very long. Some of my dishes are "one-pot meal" so they'll include different nutrients. Other dishes, like grilled chicken, should be paired with vegetables. Try to plan your meals for the day to make sure you are getting all the necessary nutrients. If you ate oatmeal for breakfast, then had brown rice with your lunch, skip the complex carbohydrates at dinner. As long as the food is "clean" -- not processed, it's suitable to eat. Use your creativity to make wonderful meals.

"People who balance their protein throughout the day, eating some at each meal, saw more weight loss or maintenance than those who skimped on the nutrient at certain meals, reports a new study analysis in the American Journal of Clinical Nutrition."

I use the phrase "food ideas" because some dishes are so easy to make, there is barely a recipe for them. But, it's a suggestion for you. It's difficult to come up with meals every day. I hope this section serves as a catalyst to create some wonderful healthy dishes on your own. When you do... share them with me. I'm always searching for new ideas!

BREAKFAST

Protein Oatmeal

Good for you! Full of fiber and helps to lower LDL (bad cholesterol)

1/3 cup old fashioned oats

2/3 cup water or almond milk

½ teaspoon vanilla extra

2 teaspoons peanut butter

½ scoop vanilla protein powder

Combine oats and water/milk in a small saucepan. Bring to a boil. Reduce heat and let oatmeal simmer. Remove from heat and add in protein powder and vanilla. Pour into bowl and stir in peanut butter.

Go to Bed Family Oatmeal (Slow Cooker Recipe)

1 cup steel cut oats

2 ½ cups almond or coconut milk

¼ cup pure maple syrup

1 cup apple, peeled and chopped

1/3 cup raisins

1/3 cup chopped walnuts and pecans

1 teaspoon cinnamon

Line slow cooker with liner or spray with cooking spray. Add all ingredients and mix well. Set dial to low and cook for 8 – 9 hours. You'll wake up in the morning to hot oatmeal, all ready to eat!

Peachy, Peanut Buttery, Brown Rice Breakfast Bowl

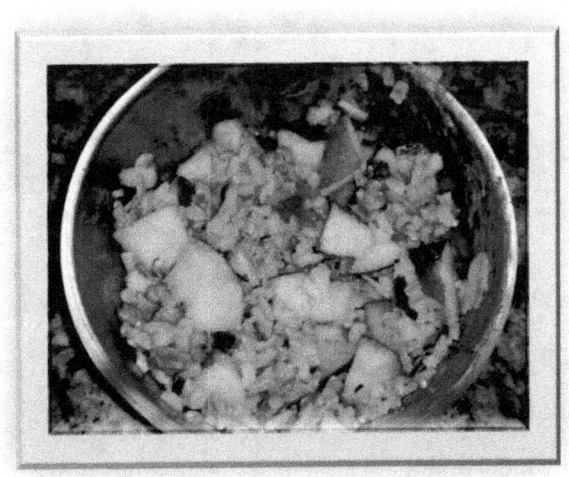

Quick and easy breakfast idea, especially if you make the rice ahead of time.

4 tablespoons brown rice

1 tablespoons sliced almonds

1 fresh peach (or any fruit)

1 teaspoon peanut butter.

Mix all ingredients together in a bowl and microwave for one minute. Enjoy!

Fruity Almond Buttery, Brown Rice Breakfast Bowl

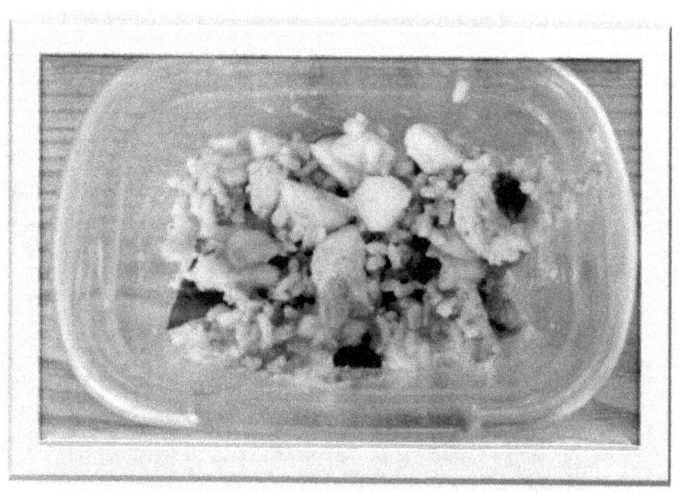

4 tablespoons brown rice

1/4 cup chopped apple

½ banana, cut into pieces

1 teaspoon almond butter

1 tablespoon cranberries & raisins

1 tablespoon walnuts, chopped

Sprinkle of cinnamon

Mix all ingredients together in a bowl and microwave for 1 minute. It's ready!

Protein Pancakes

1 egg

¼ cup steel cut oats

½ scoop vanilla protein powder

Coconut oil

Mix steel cut oats with egg. Stir and add protein powder. Coat a skillet with coconut oil. Once the oil gets hot, pour batter. Turn pancake over once. Cook until golden brown.

Banana Pancakes

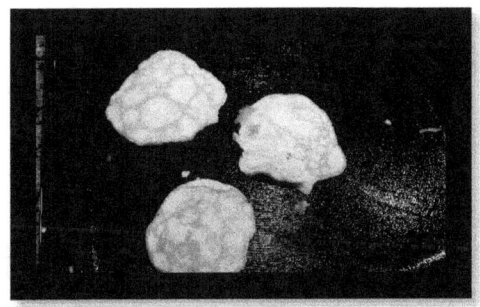

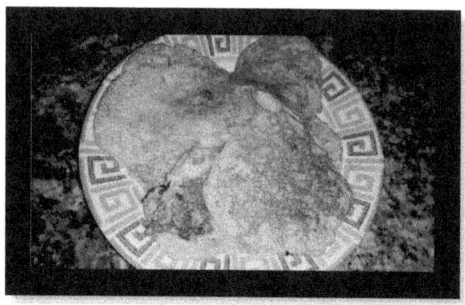

These are easy and one of my favorites in the morning.

1 banana

2 eggs

Cinnamon

Pumpkin pie spice

Mash one banana in a small bowl. In a separate bowl, whisk two eggs. Mix together and sprinkle with cinnamon and pumpkin pie spice. Coat the skillet with coconut oil. Once the oil gets hot, pour batter. Turn pancake over once. Cook until golden brown. The batter is thin so they cook quickly.

All About Eggs

Eggs have gotten a bad rap in the past but recent research, shows that eggs are not associated with "bad" cholesterol the way we once thought. The cholesterol you eat has little impact on the amount of cholesterol in our blood. Your body makes cholesterol on its own (about 1 and 2 grams) and it is largely determined by genetics, exercise and stress levels. We do need some cholesterol, as it is an important nutrient for growth and the production of many hormones. That means you can eat the whole egg. Eggs contain six grams of easily-absorbed protein and are only 76 calories. The yolk contains lutein and zeaxanthin, major antioxidants that help prevent eye diseases, and choline, which is needed for brain development in a growing fetus and for brain function in adults.

In addition, eggs are rich in Vitamin D -- important for bones and teeth. It also aids in the absorption of calcium. If you are only eating the whites, you are missing out on many of the key nutrients. Recent studies have found that people who ate eggs for breakfast consumed 330 fewer calories throughout the day than those who had a carbohydrate rich breakfast, like a bagel.

Of course, if you have diabetes or hypercholesterolemia (a high level of cholesterol in your blood), don't eat the yolk. However, if you have normal levels and your diet is relatively healthy, eat the whole egg. Personally, I do eat the yolks but decide what's best for you.

Hard Boiled Eggs

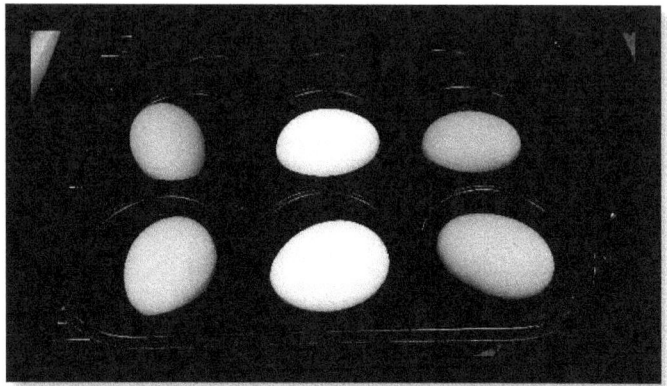

Keep hard-boiled eggs in the house. Add them to salads, have them for breakfast, bring them to work or eat one before you exercise for a quick protein fix. I know stores now offer pre-made hard boiled eggs. I've tried them, but they taste a little "funny" to me. I prefer to make a batch of my own in the beginning of the week. A shortcut only works if it's good.

(My dog Lola absolutely loves the yolk. No matter where she is in the house, she can hear me crack the egg and runs to get her treat.)

Scrambled Eggs with Peppers, Cheese & Chia Seeds

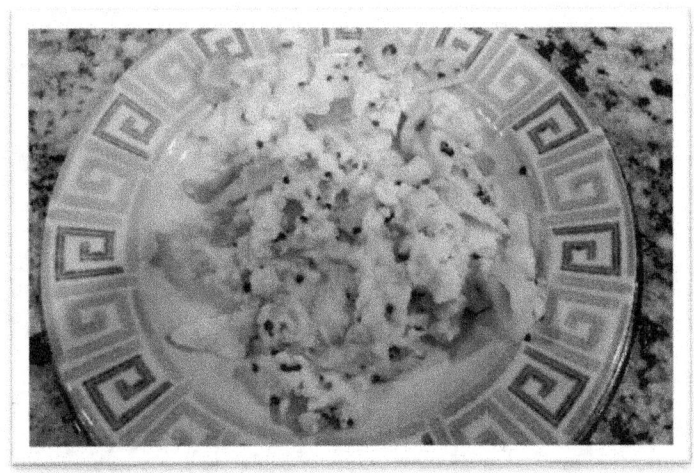

Scrambled eggs are great and easy to make that even my son can cook them now. Mix them with veggies like tomatoes, zucchini, mushrooms, broccoli and spinach. Or make an omelet and put veggies inside.

2 eggs
2 mini peppers, sliced
2 tablespoons shredded mozzarella cheese
Sprinkle of chia seeds

Spray a small pan with cooking spray. Whisk eggs in a bowl and add peppers. Mix well. Cook on heated pan. Add mozzarella and chia seeds at the end of cooking.

Eggs and Brown Rice

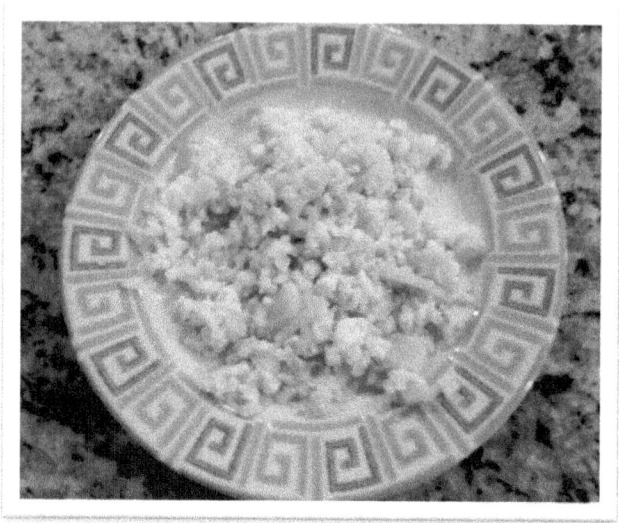

2 eggs

2 tablespoons brown rice

Half a chopped yellow pepper

Sprinkle of fresh parmesan cheese

Spray a small pan with cooking spray. Whisk eggs in a separate bowl and add brown rice and peppers. Mix well. Cook on heated pan. Add parmesan at the end of cooking.

Eggs and Kale

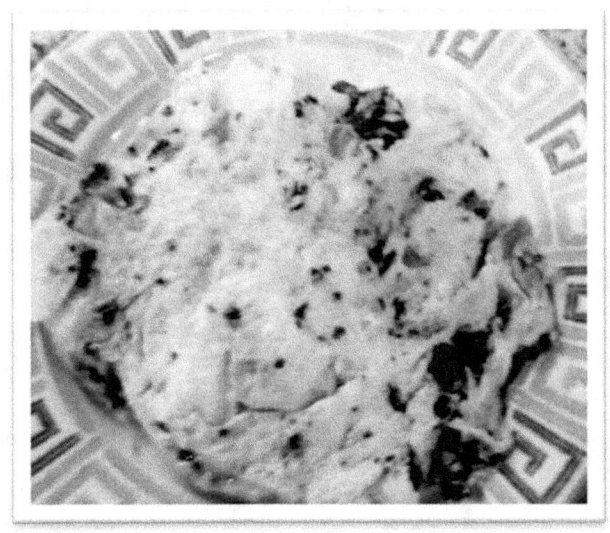

2 eggs

½ cup kale, chopped

Sprinkle of fresh parmesan cheese

Spray a small pan with cooking spray. Whisk eggs in a separate bowl and add kale. Mix well. Cook on heated pan. Add parmesan at the end of cooking.

Muffin Tin Eggs

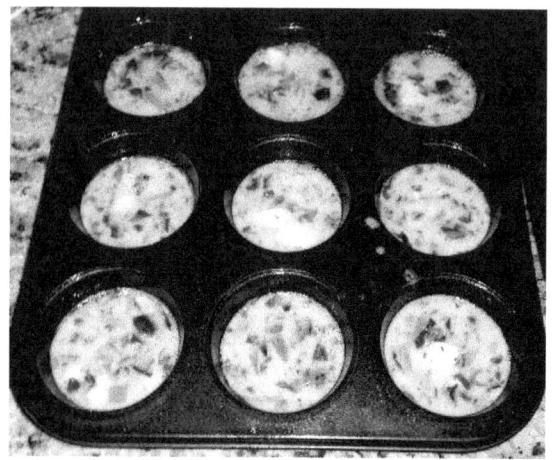

Another easy way to eat eggs is: mix them with veggies and put them in muffin tins. These provide instant portion control and will keep them in the refrigerator for a few days. Depending on their size, have 1 or 2 for breakfast, especially on those hectic days.

6 large eggs

Broccoli, chopped

Spinach

½ onion

Grated cheese

Mix the eggs, veggies onion and cheese in a bowl. Spray the tins first with cooking spray. Pour egg mixture into muffin tins and bake at 350 degrees for approximately 20 minutes.

Spinach Pie

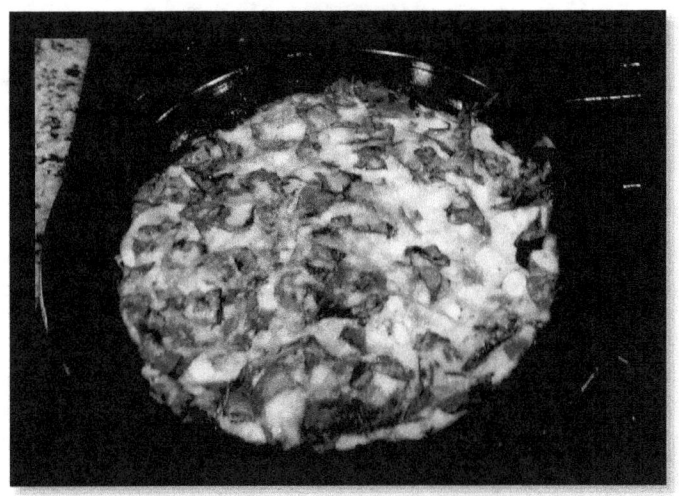

If you aren't a fan of a typical breakfast, try this. Make ahead of time and just cut a piece for breakfast. It can also be used as a side dish at meals too.

3 eggs

About 6-7 ounces of fresh spinach, chopped

1/2 cup + 2 tablespoons cottage cheese

2 sprinkles of light cheddar cheese

Chopped onion

Garlic & pepper to taste

Mix together all ingredients. Spray a pie plate or lightly coat with olive oil. Spread mixture into plate. Bake at 350 degrees for approximately 45 minutes.

Cottage Cheese Spice

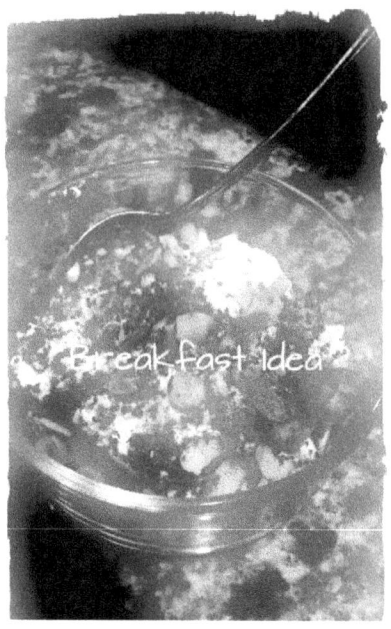

Full of protein and low on calories.

Low-fat cottage cheese

Apples, pears, bananas

Sliced almonds

Chia seeds

Pumpkin pie spice

Cinnamon

Honey (if desired)

Cut up fruit and mix with cottage cheese. Sprinkle almonds, spices, chia seeds (and honey). Enjoy!

Pumpkin Yogurt

A simple idea -- especially if you're a pumpkin lover.

1 cup vanilla yogurt (low in sugar)

½ cup pumpkin puree

1/2 teaspoon cinnamon

1 teaspoon pumpkin pie spice

Mix pumpkin with vanilla yogurt. Add cinnamon, pumpkin pie spice and sliced almonds. Delicious!

Almond Milk Protein Shake

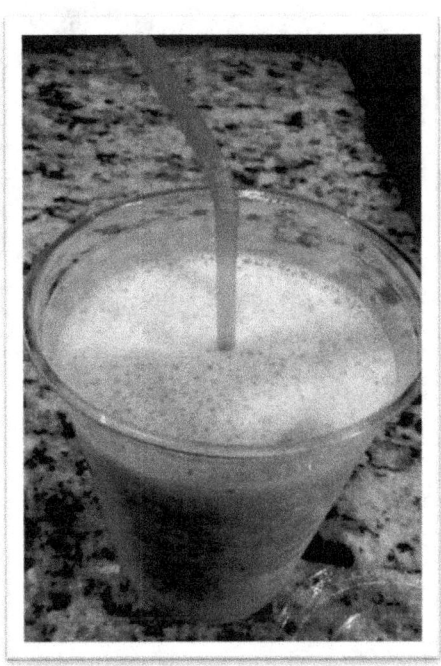

I love protein shakes in the morning or after a workout.

1 banana – fresh or frozen

1 cup almond milk

1 scoop vanilla protein powder

Sprinkle of cinnamon

Ice

Additional Options: ½ cup pumpkin, 1 teaspoon peanut butter, various berries

Using a blender, mix all ingredients together. Drink with a straw.

Coconut Milk Protein Shake

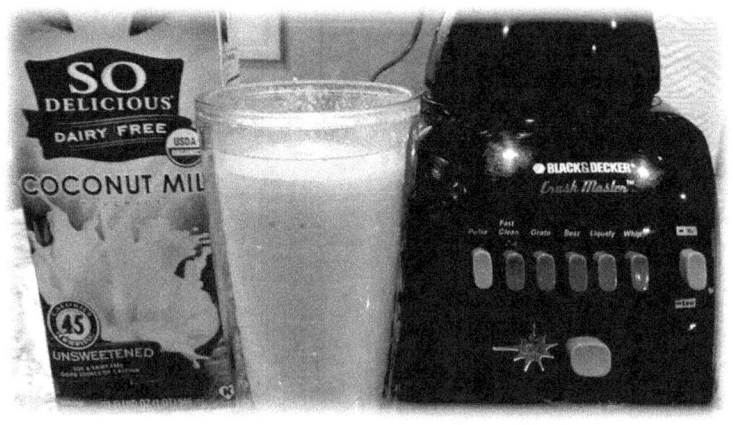

½ banana – fresh or frozen

1 cup coconut milk

1 scoop vanilla protein powder

Frozen pineapple pieces

1 teaspoon peanut butter

Dash of banana extra (can substitute vanilla extract)

Ice

Using a blender, mix all ingredients together. Drink with a straw.

Chocolate Protein Shake

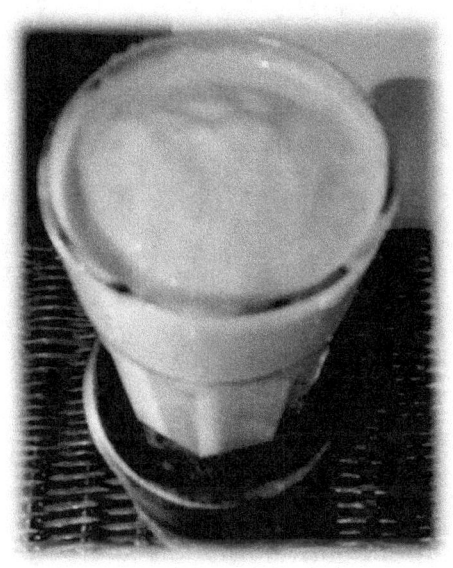

It may seem strange to add avocado but it makes the shake so creamy. My son said it tasted just like a chocolate milk shake.

1 banana – fresh or frozen

1 cup almond milk

1 scoop chocolate protein powder

½ medium avocado

Ice

Using a blender, mix all ingredients together. Drink with a straw.

Nuts & Fruit Granola

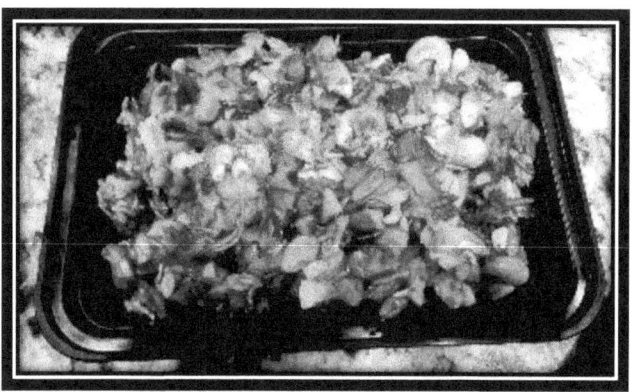

Many store-bought kinds have a lot of sugar so I started making my own. For this recipe, I pretty much put whatever I have in the house at the time. And I don't measure!

Approximately 1 cup old fashioned oats

Walnuts

Pecans

Almonds

Mix the ingredients in a bowl with a little bit of honey, a touch of pure maple syrup, cinnamon, and pumpkin pie spice. Spread on a cookie sheet lined with parchment paper and bake in a preheated oven at 400 degrees for about 10 minutes. After 10 minutes, add 1 or 2 of the following ingredients and bake for another 5 minutes:

Dates

Raisins

Coconut

Cranberries

Sunflower seeds

Let it cool, put in airtight containers and enjoy!

Hazelnut Granola

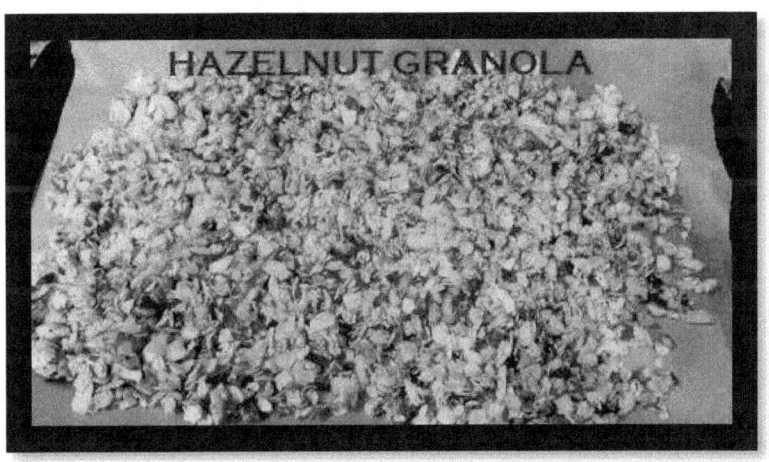

1 cup old fashioned oats

1 cup chopped hazelnuts

1/2 cup sliced almonds

1/2 cup unsweetened shredded coconut

1/4 cup honey

Preheat oven to 350 degrees. Mix all ingredients together and bake for approximately 20-25 minutes. Toss once or twice while baking to prevent burning.

Pumpkin Granola Bars

These bars are good for a quick breakfast in the morning. Or a snack anytime.

1 ½ cups quick cooking oats

½ cup pumpkin

½ cup unsweetened apple sauce

1 cup peanut butter

1/3 cup honey

1 scoop vanilla protein powder

2 teaspoons pumpkin pie spice

1 teaspoon cinnamon

Preheat oven to 350 degrees. Roast oats for 10-15 minutes on a cookie sheet (nice golden brown color.) Cool completely. Mix all ingredients together in a bowl. Spread onto a raised cookie sheet or baking dish – ½ inch thick. Bake for 20 minutes. Cool and slice into bars. Store in an airtight container.

VEGETABLES

Roasted Vegetables

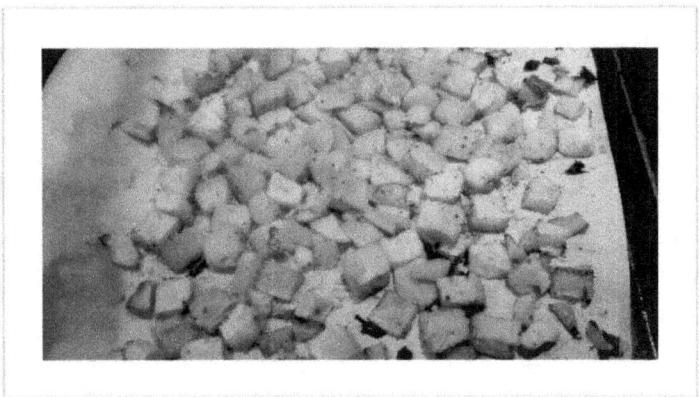

Butternut Squash

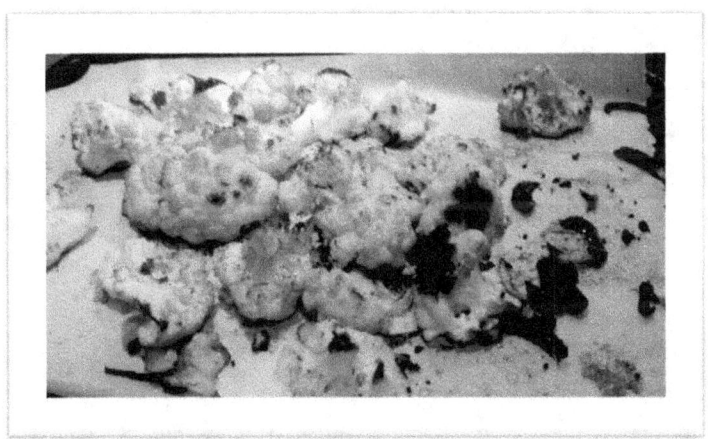

Cauliflower

I love to roast fresh vegetables right in the oven. Use as a side dish or a snack. This can be done with lots of different veggies:

Asparagus

Cauliflower

Broccoli

Brussel Sprouts

String beans

Squash

Cut up veggies and put into a bowl. Drizzle olive oil on them, not too much, but enough to moisten. Add seasonings, like lemon pepper, garlic, onion powder and even some grated cheese. Roast in a preheated oven at 425 degrees for approximately 15 minutes.

Sautéed Kale

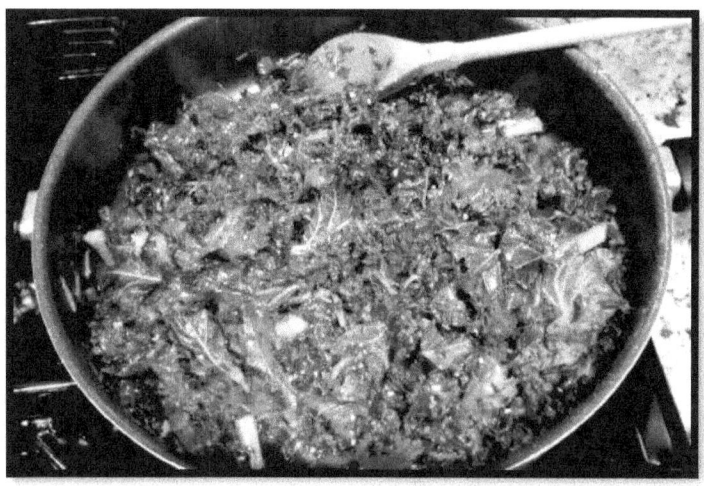

One of the healthiest vegetables - full of Vitamins C, A and K.

2 bunches of kale, rinsed and dried, stems removed

2 tablespoons olive oil

2 cloves garlic

Ground black pepper

In a large skillet, heat the oil over medium heat. Sauté the garlic. Add kale and toss to coat with oil. Put the lid on and cover for approximately 5 minutes. Remove lid, season with pepper.

Kale Chips

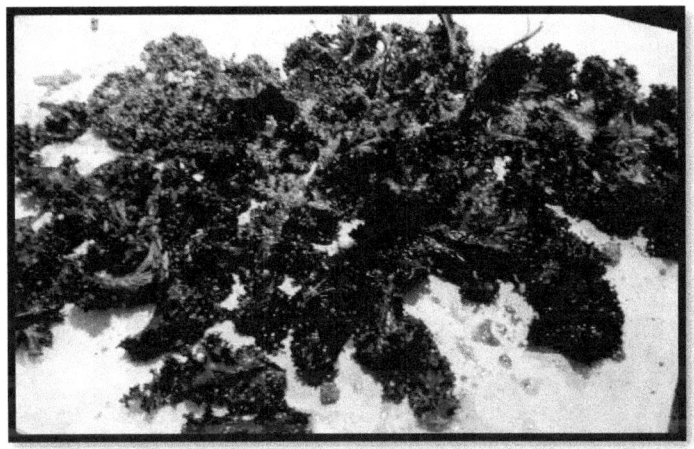

Looking for a crunchy, healthy snack? Try kale chips - they are so easy to make. These are a great alternative to potato chips. They taste good and can be quite addictive.

Kale, rinsed and dried, stems removed

Olive oil

Various spices (I use no-salt lemon pepper.)

Parmesan cheese

Pull the leaves off the thick stem of the kale. Put the kale leaves in a bowl and drizzle with olive oil. Add spices and mix well. Lay the leaves flat on a cookie sheet. Bake in a 350 degree oven until crispy, about 10-15 minutes.

Baked Tomatoes

Tomatoes, sliced

4 teaspoons olive oil

1 teaspoon Italian spices

Fresh basil

Parmesan cheese

Fresh pepper

Preheat oven to 400 degrees. Place tomatoes on a baking sheet. Drizzle olive oil and sprinkle the rest of the ingredients on top of each slice. Bake for about 15 minutes.

Sweet Potatoes

I love sweet potato. They are so versatile. The simplest way to eat them -- just bake in the oven or, even better, on an outdoor grill. Don't add butter -- you don't need it. They are excellent plain.

Sweet Potato (Chips)

A great way to eat sweet potatoes: chips!

Sweet potato

Olive oil, enough to cover

Garlic powder

Ground black pepper

Use a mandolin or food processor to slice the potatoes very thin. Put them in a bowl with olive oil and spices. Put on a baking sheet and bake in a preheated 425 degree oven until crispy. *Note – instead of the garlic powder and pepper, try adding some cinnamon to make them a sweet treat.*

Fresh Veggie Mix

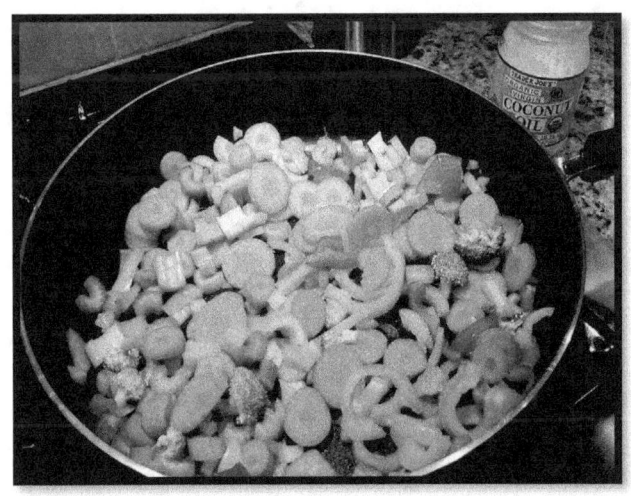

Quick, easy and fresh!

Carrots

Celery

Onions

Peppers

Coconut oil

Cut up veggies. In a large skillet, sauté onions and peppers with coconut oil. Add carrots and celery. Add a little water and put lid on for approximately 10 minutes. Cook until tender.

Spaghetti Squash

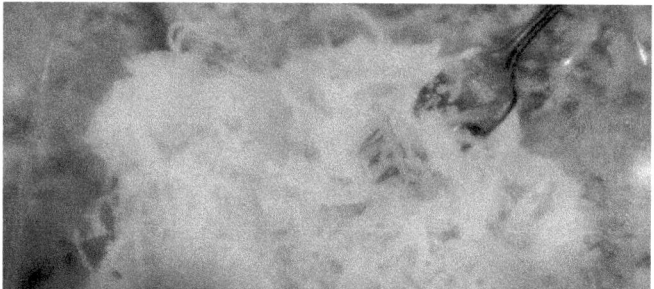

A wonderful alternative to pasta. Two ways to cook the squash – boiling or baking:

(1) Pierce holes in the squash and boil in a pot full of water. Once it comes to a rolling boil, put on the lid and cook until tender, approximately 25 minutes

(2) Pierce holes in the squash and place in a preheated oven – 375

degrees. Bake until squash has softened.

For both methods - let it cool, then cut the squash in half. Scoop out the seeds that are in the middle of the squash. Using a fork, begin to scrape the insides of the squash and you will see "spaghetti" start to form.

Mix in your favorite healthy sauce and eat as is. Or, try some pesto and lightly sauté it with fresh veggies like broccoli and carrots. Add in some chicken sausage or shrimp. Make a casserole by adding crumbled meatballs (93% lean meat), mixed in with light ricotta cheese, marinara sauce and some parmesan. Bake for about 20 minutes.

Veggie Jumble

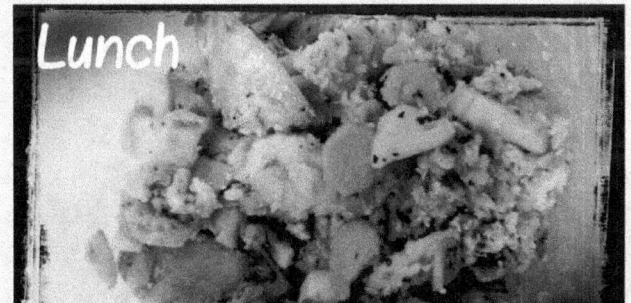

I made this for lunch one day. I used whatever I had in the refrigerator and it came out really good so now I make it on purpose.

Carrots, cut up

Turnips, sliced

Sweet potato, chopped into small pieces

Veggie burger*

Coconut Oil

* There are many different kinds of veggie burgers out there. Since I'm not looking for a meat substitute, I choose ones with lots of veggies and a high protein content.

Heat coconut oil in a large skillet. Add carrots, turnips and sweet potato. Sauté and put lid on to soften up veggies. Add veggie burger and break into pieces while stirring. Serve warm.

Carrot Coconut Bites

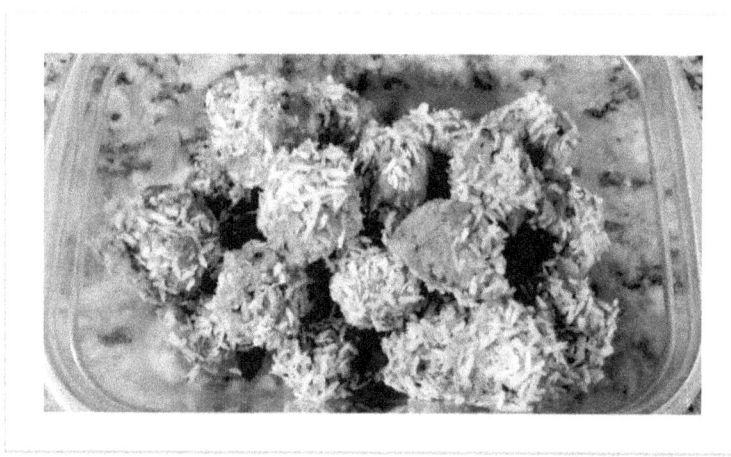

I put this recipe under vegetables but it's not a dinner side dish. It's really a snack made out of carrots. My son loves them. They don't look "pretty" but they taste really good.

4 carrots, washed & peeled

¾ cup nuts (I've used almonds, pecans, hazelnuts – whatever I had in the house – pick one!)

1 cup unsweetened coconut

4 dried figs (Add more or less for your individual taste.)

2 dates – (Can be omitted.)

¼ cup honey (Note: if you use dates – use a little less honey.)

Cinnamon

Shred the carrots. (I use a food processor with a shred blade.) After the carrots are shredded, put all ingredients in a food processor, except ½ cup of coconut. (Reserve for later.) Blend it together for approximately 1-2 minutes. The mixture should be thick enough to handle. Form small balls and roll into reserved coconut. Refrigerate for a few hours or overnight.

SOUPS

I love making soups because they are easy to make, they're filling, and can be a healthy option for a meal.

Mexican Chicken Soup

1 tablespoon olive oil

1 small onion

1 jalapeno pepper, diced

1 clove garlic

5 cups low sodium chicken broth

1 ½ lbs boneless, skinless chicken breasts, cut into strips

1 ½ cups mild salsa

1 teaspoon cumin

1 teaspoon chili powder

Pepper, to taste

Heat oil in a large pot over medium heat. Add onion and jalapeno pepper. Cook until tender, about 5 minutes. Stir in garlic and spices. Increase heat and add broth. Bring to a boil. Add chicken and cook until no longer pink. Stir in salsa, season with pepper and simmer for 10 minutes.

Veggie Soup

4 teaspoon olive oil

1 medium onion, diced

1 clove garlic

Broccoli

Carrots

Celery

Spinach

Any other fresh veggies you like

(Note: Cut up vegetables will equal about 4 cups. Variety depends on availability and preference.)

4 cups organic low sodium vegetable or chicken broth

Fresh pepper

Heat olive oil in a large pot. Sauté onions and garlic on medium heat. Add all other vegetables and season with pepper. Add broth and bring soup to a boil. Reduce heat to low. Put lid on and simmer for approximately 30 minutes.

Roasted Vegetable Soup

This one is super easy! It uses leftover roasted vegetables (see Roasted Veggies recipe).

Oven roasted vegetables
3-4 cups organic low sodium vegetable or chicken broth
2 % or skim milk (optional)

In a large saucepan, mix vegetables and broth. Heat on medium and simmer for approximately 10 minutes. Put mixture into a blender and puree. Pour soup back into saucepan. If using milk, add a few splashes for a creamier texture. If you like a thinner consistency soup, add more broth or some water. Reheat if necessary.

Carrot, Apple Ginger Soup

4 cups chopped, peeled carrots
3 tablespoons olive oil
1 clove garlic
1 small onion, chopped
2 tablespoons fresh ginger, peeled and grated
1 small apple

4 cups organic low-sodium vegetable broth

Pinch of nutmeg

Fresh pepper

Garlic powder

2 % or skim milk (optional)

Boil carrots until soft. Peel an apple and cut into little pieces. Heat olive oil in a large pot on medium heat. Sauté an onion and some fresh ginger for about one minute. Mix the carrots, apples, onion and ginger with vegetable stock. Heat until it boils. Add some garlic powder, a touch of nutmeg and pepper. Using an immersion blender, blend everything together (or pour into a blender.) Add a splash of milk, if desired. Blend soup to suit your desired consistency – thick or thin. Season to taste with a touch of nutmeg, pepper and garlic powder.

Pumpkin Soup

2 cups pumpkin puree – homemade (see recipe below) or organic canned

2 tablespoons olive oil

1 small onion

2 tablespoons fresh ginger, peeled and grated

4 cups low-sodium chicken broth

Pepper to taste

Heat oil in a large pot. Add onions and cook until translucent. Add pumpkin, ginger and low-sodium chicken broth and bring to a boil. Use an immersion blender or regular blender to your desired consistency. Return to pot and season with pepper.

Pumpkin Puree

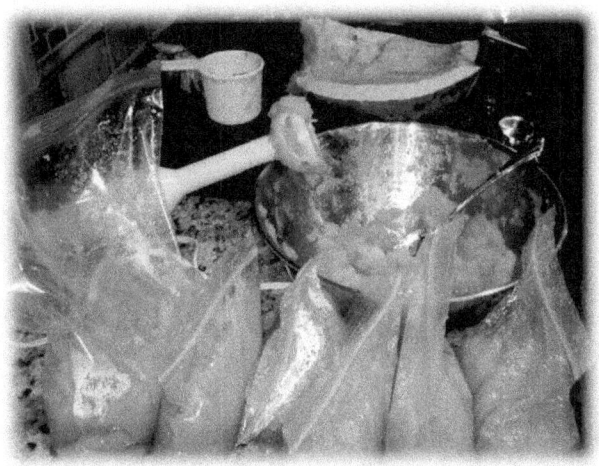

I love pumpkin! Whenever I see a recipe with it, I have to try it. I live on the East coast so during the fall, pumpkin is everywhere. I usually buy a few and make homemade puree. I measure out portions by cups. Put it into baggies and freeze them. This way, I always have fresh pumpkin (as opposed to canned) throughout the year.

Sugar Pumpkins are best for cooking. Preheat oven to 350 degrees. Line a baking sheet with parchment paper. Cut the tops off pumpkins and halve them. Scoop out the "meat," seeds and strings. Save the seeds for roasting later. Place face down on the baking sheet and bake for 45-50 minutes. A fork should easily pierce the skin. Remove from oven and let cool. Peel skin and put pumpkin in a blender. Measure and place in baggies to freeze for future recipes.

Roasted Pumpkin Seeds

Seeds (reserved from puree recipe)
Olive oil to coat
Fresh pepper (salt, if desired)

Preheat the oven to 400 degrees. Rinse the seeds and dry them well. Once dry, put the seeds in a bowl with olive oil and spices. Mix well. Line a baking sheet with parchment paper in a single layer. Bake for approximately 10 minutes. Once the seeds turn a light brown, they're done.

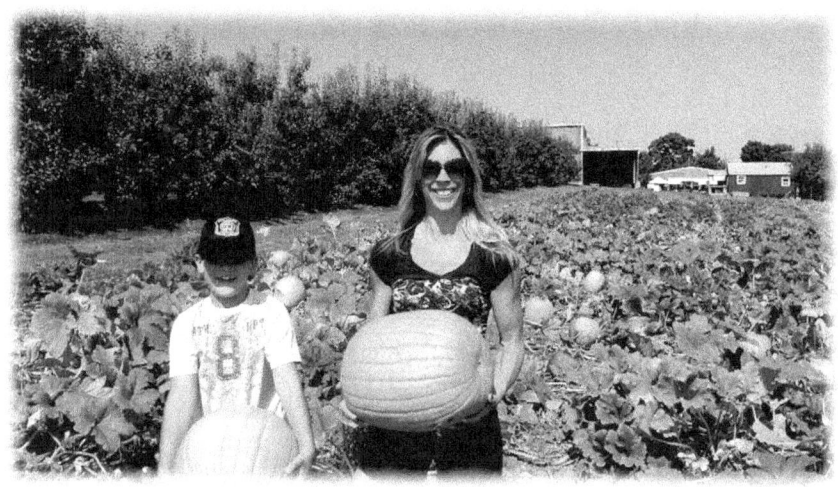

Pumpkin Picking
Had to get a big one – I love Pumpkin!

SALADS

Cucumber Tomato Salad

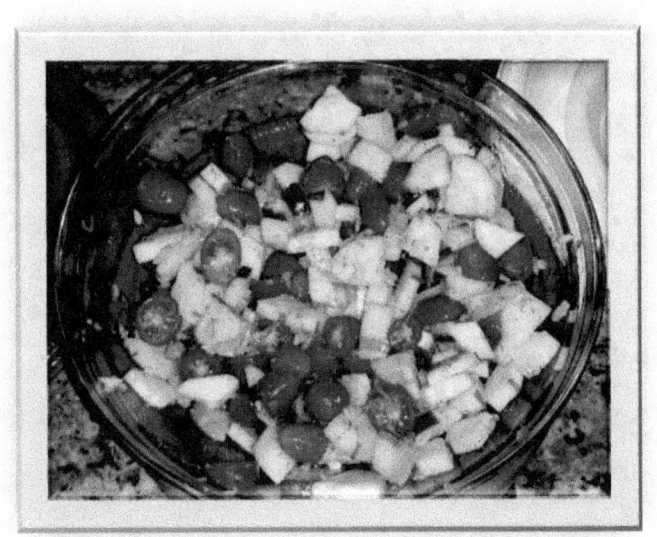

2 whole cucumbers

½ pint grape tomatoes

½ red onion

Fresh herbs *(I use basil, oregano and basil from my garden.)*

Touch of extra virgin olive oil

Dice cucumbers. Halve tomatoes. Chop onion finely. Mix all ingredients together in a bowl, adding olive oil to cover.

Spinach Salad

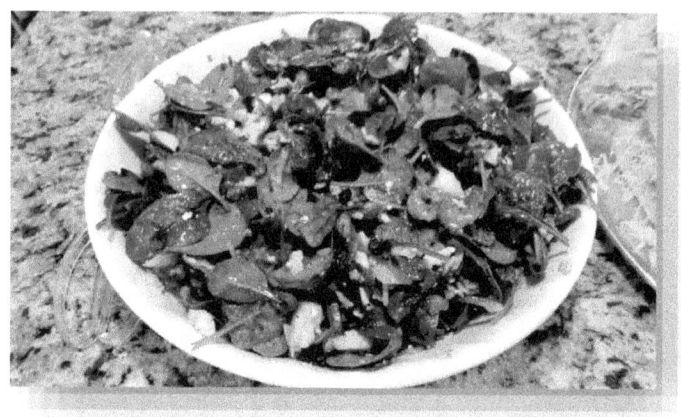

Organic baby spinach

1 large pear, cut up

Reduced-fat Feta cheese

Cranberries

Chopped pecans

Dressing: juice of 1/2 lemon, 1/4 teaspoon honey, 1/4 cup olive oil, pepper to taste

Mix all ingredients in a large bowl. Make dressing in a separate bowl and pour over salad. Toss and serve.

Cobb Salad

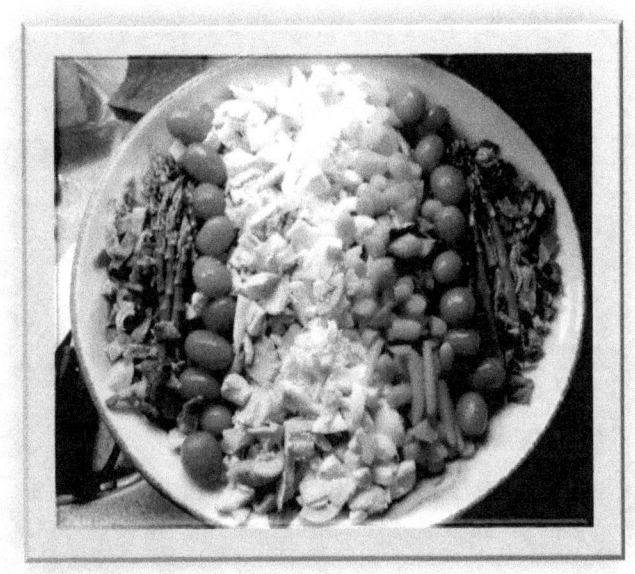

Chicken breast, chopped and cooked

Carrots

Hard boiled eggs, sliced

Grape tomatoes, whole

Asparagus, blanched

Bacon *(Note: Since the salad is divided by ingredients, it's easy to just take a taste of the bacon. A little bite is okay for flavor. Don't grab spoonfuls of it.)*

Dressing:

3 tablespoons white wine vinegar

1 tablespoon extra virgin olive oil

Italian seasonings

121

Separate each ingredient and place in sections on a large plate. Make the dressing in a separate bowl and pour over salad. Ready to serve!

Grilled Asparagus Salad

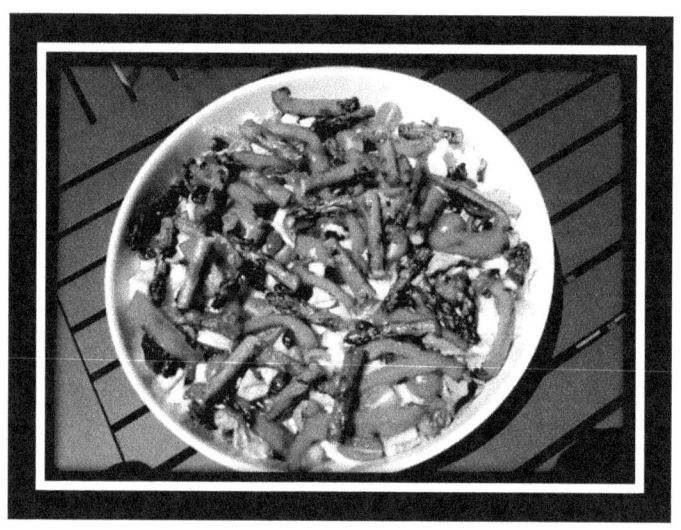

Asparagus, grilled

Red peppers, cut into strips

Greek olives

Romaine lettuce

Grape tomatoes, halved

Diced cucumbers

Dressing:

Extra virgin olive oil

Balsamic vinegar

Layer ingredients in a large bowl, lettuce, tomatoes, cucumbers, olives, red peppers and asparagus. Make the dressing in a separate bowl and pour over salad.

Sweet Salad

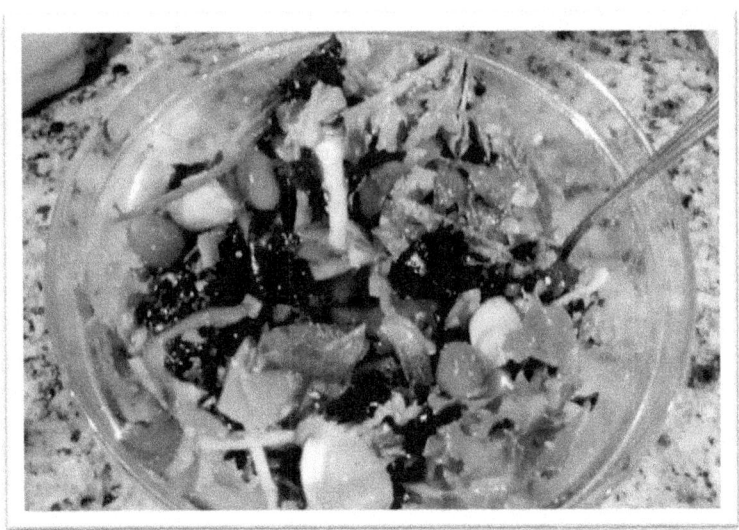

Romaine lettuce

Tomatoes

Sweet peppers

Squash, cut into pieces

Carrots, sliced

Grated parmesan cheese

Dressing:

Extra virgin olive oil

1/2 lemon

1 teaspoon of honey

Fresh herbs - oregano, basil & cilantro.

Mix all ingredients in a large bowl. Make the dressing in a separate bowl and add together. Toss and serve.

CAT (Corn, Avocado, Tomato) Salad

2 cups corn (fresh is best but can substitute frozen)

1 avocado, diced

1 pint cherry tomatoes

1 small red onion, diced

2 tablespoons olive oil

1 tablespoon juice of lime

¼ cup chopped cilantro

Fresh ground pepper, to taste

In a large bowl, whisk together the olive oil, lime juice, cilantro and pepper. Mix in the corn, avocado, tomatoes and onion.

Arugula Fig Salad

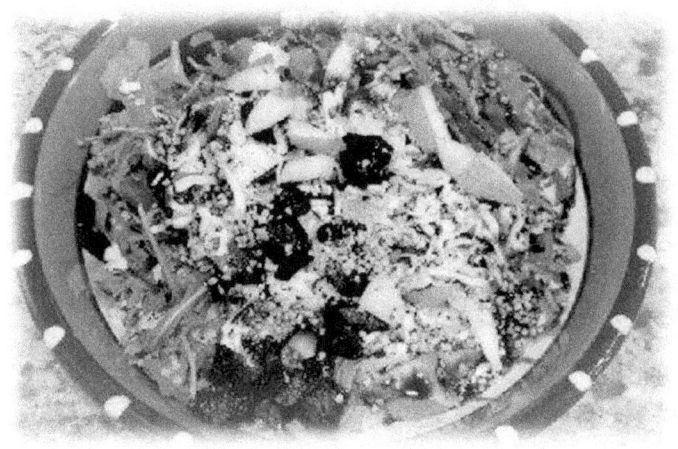

Arugula

Sun dried tomatoes

Turkey slices

Fresh mozzarella, cut into pieces

½ pear, cut into pieces

4 figs, cut into pieces

1 tablespoon hemp hearts

Dressing:

Extra virgin olive oil

Balsamic vinegar

Mix all ingredients together in a large bowl. Add vinegar and oil.
Toss and serve.

Crab Avocado Salad

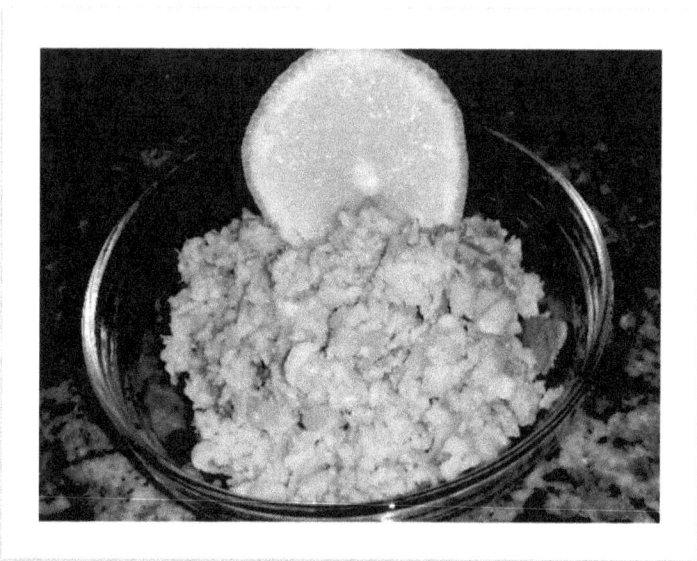

1 medium avocado

4 oz. soft crab meat

½ red onion, finely chopped

2 celery stalks, finely chopped

1 teaspoon extra virgin olive oil

Juice of 1 lemon (or lime)

Fresh pepper

In a medium bowl, combine olive oil, lime juice, onion and pepper. Add crab meat. Cut avocado in half and spoon out avocado into bowl. Be careful not to mash the avocado. Gently stir and serve.

Chicken Salad

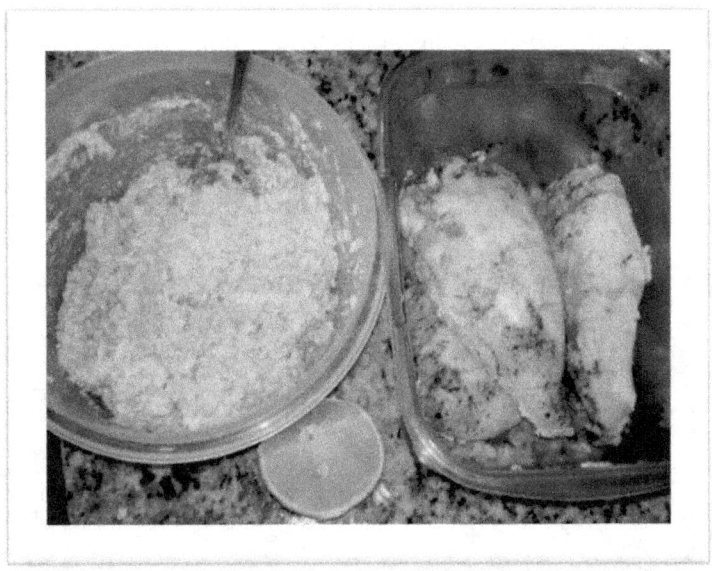

Chicken breasts, cooked (Chicken can be made ahead by baking in the oven.)

Carrots, finely chopped

Celery, chopped

Cranberries

Walnuts, chopped

Grapes, cut in half

1 small onion

1 tablespoon low fat or light mayo

½ juice of lemon

Garlic powder

Fresh pepper

Mix chicken, carrots, celery, and onion with mayo in food processor. Transfer to large bowl and add lemon, garlic powder and pepper. Mix in cranberries, walnuts and grapes. Stir and serve.

Fruit Salad

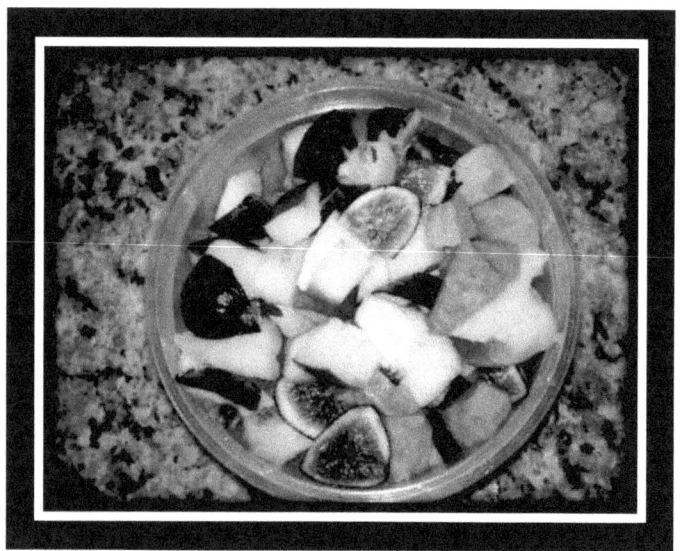

This sounds so simple but I add it here as more of a reminder. Sometimes you don't feel like eating a whole apple. But you might like it better if the fruit was already cut up. Make a fruit salad using fresh fruit. In the summer, use the berries – strawberries, blueberries, raspberries. Or melons – watermelon, cantaloupe and honeydew. In the winter, use apples, bananas and pears. If fresh fruit isn't available, buy a bag of frozen fruit and throw it in a bowl. It doesn't get any easier than that.

ONE POT MEALS

I like the idea of everything being in just one pot. It's easy, quick and versatile. One pot meals can be made into Mexican fiestas, Asian stir-frys, and Italian night.

Turkey Time Dish

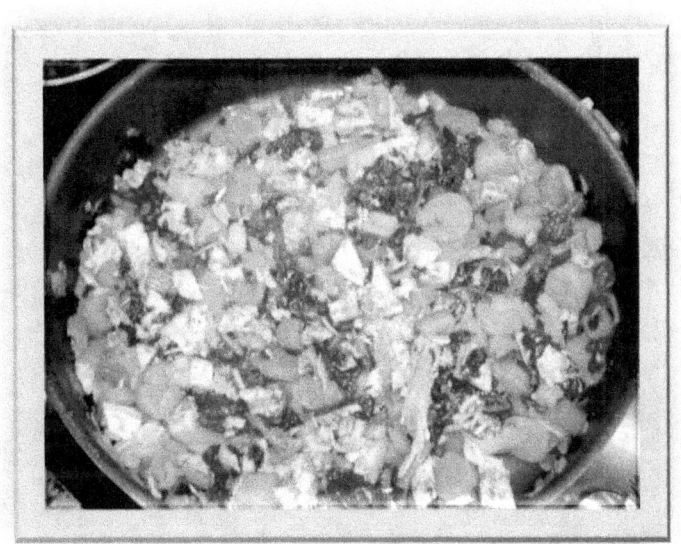

Turkey (leftovers)

1 small onion, chopped

1 cup celery, chopped

1 cup carrots, chopped

3-4 cups kale

1 clove garlic

3 tablespoons olive oil

Low sodium soy sauce

Ginger

Heat olive oil on medium heat in a 3-qt. covered sauté pan. Cook onion and garlic. Add veggies and cook until softened. Mix in cooked turkey and add low sodium soy sauce and ginger. Put cover on and simmer for approximately 15 minutes. Stir and serve.

Quick Chicken & Veggies

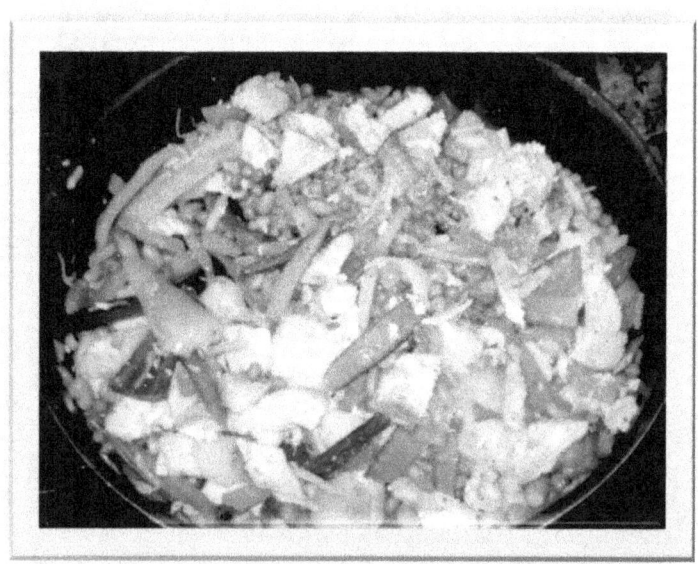

This recipe uses chicken that was cooked ahead of time and frozen veggies. Fresh is best but in a pinch, frozen is fine.

Grilled chicken (cooked ahead of time)

Sugar snap peas

Peppers

Bag of frozen veggies (carrots, peas, lima beans)

Olive oil

Low sodium soy sauce

Ginger paste or fresh ginger (peeled & cut)

Juice of a lime

Heat olive oil on medium heat in a 3-qt. covered sauté pan. Add veggies and cook until softened. Mix in cooked chicken and add low sodium soy sauce and ginger. Put cover on and simmer for approximately 15 minutes. Stir and serve.

Mediterranean Chicken

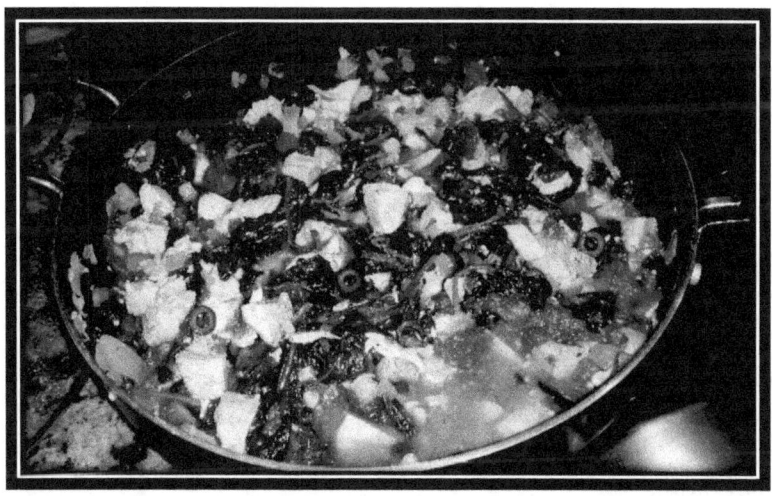

Chicken breasts, cut into pieces

2-3 cups fresh spinach *(It shrinks.)*

1 onion, chopped

2 cloves garlic

1 small can of black olives

1 can whole peeled tomato

½ cup white wine

½ cup chicken broth

Olive oil

Heat oil on medium heat in a 3-quart covered sauté pan. Brown chicken breast in olive oil. Add onions, garlic and olives. Cook for approximately 5 minutes. Add spinach, wine and broth. Cover the pan and reduce to low heat. Let simmer then serve.

Mexican Chicken Dish

Extra virgin olive oil

Chicken tenderloins

Salsa

Sweet peppers, cut into slices

Edamame

Corn

Black beans

Black olives, sliced

1 small onion

1 clove garlic

Chili powder

Pepper

Tortilla chips (for garnish)

Heat olive oil on medium heat in a 3-qt. covered sauté pan. Cook onion and garlic. Add chicken and cook until it's no longer pink. Mix in sweet peppers, corn, edamame, olives, black beans and salsa. Stir and add chili powder and pepper. Put lid on and simmer for approximately 15 minutes. Stir and serve. Add a couple of tortilla chips on top for crunch.

Mexican Shrimp Dish

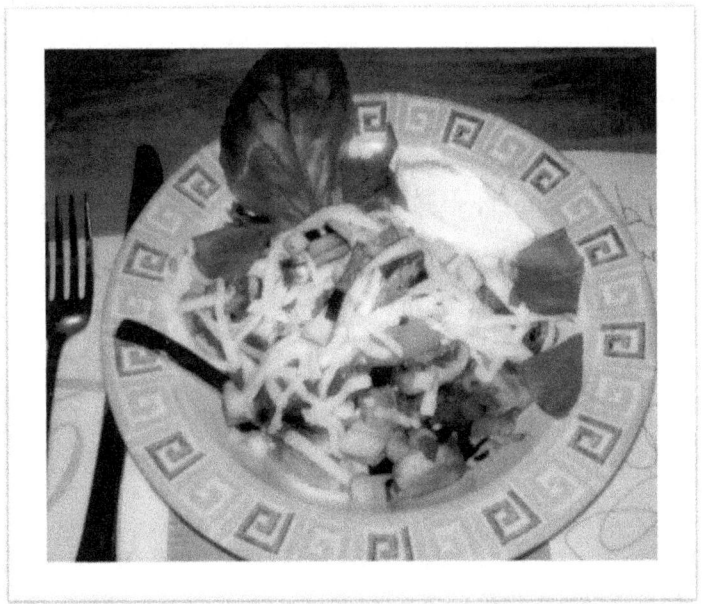

1 lb. medium shrimp

1 small onion

1 small package fresh mushrooms

1 green pepper

1 yellow pepper

1 clove garlic

2 tablespoons olive oil

Chopped cilantro

Fresh basil leaves

Fresh chopped tomatoes

Low fat Mexican cheese

Dollop of light sour cream

Spoonful of salsa

In a 3-quart sauté pan, cook onions, mushrooms, green and yellow peppers, and garlic with a small amount of olive oil. Add fresh chopped cilantro and basil, fresh diced tomatoes and then add the shrimp. Simmer until shrimp are cooked through. Serve with a sprinkle of low fat Mexican cheese and a dollop of light sour cream and salsa

Seafood Dish

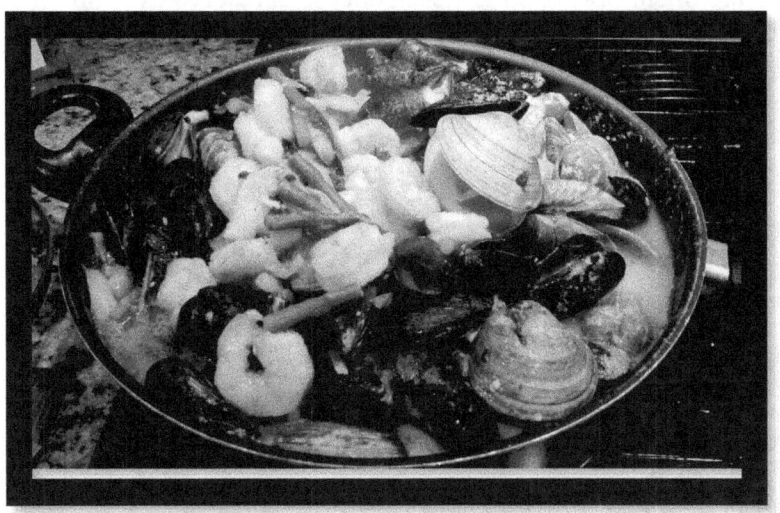

1 package of little neck clams

1 package of mussels

1 lb. of medium shrimp

1 package of bay scallops

½ lb. asparagus

¾ cups white wine

3/4 cups low sodium chicken broth

3 tablespoons olive oil

2 cloves garlic

1 small onion

Fresh parmesan cheese

Heat olive oil on medium heat in a 3-qt. covered sauté pan. Cook onion and garlic. Add chicken broth and white wine. Put in the rest of the ingredients and simmer on low heat until shrimp are pink and clams are open. Sprinkle parmesan cheese and serve over brown rice or quinoa.

Italian Meal

93% lean ground beef

1 Eggplant, cut into small pieces

2 Zucchini, cut into pieces

1 onion

2 cloves garlic

3 tablespoons olive oil

1 can crushed tomatoes

Black olives, sliced

Grape tomatoes, cut in half

Italian seasonings

Parmesan cheese

Heat olive oil on medium heat in a 3-qt. covered sauté pan. Cook onion and garlic. Set aside and cook beef. Using a colander, drain beef and return to sauté pan. Add eggplant, zucchini, olives, tomatoes and crushed tomatoes. Stir and add Italian seasonings. Put lid on and simmer for approximately 15 minutes. Sprinkle parmesan cheese on top.

Chili Chill Out

1 large onion, finely chopped

3 cloves garlic

1 green bell pepper

3 jalapeno peppers, seeds removed

2 lbs. 93% lean ground beef *or* turkey

2 large cans crushed tomatoes

1 large can tomato puree

1 can kidney or black beans, drained

1 package fresh sliced mushrooms

1 small can sliced black olives

1 bunch fresh cilantro, chopped

Sprinkle of Mexican cheese

Chili Seasoning

Chili Powder

Garlic Powder

Cumin

Cayenne pepper (if desired)

Brown beef with chili seasoning. Drain and add onion, garlic, peppers, mushrooms, and olives to beef mixture. Add tomatoes, chili powder, cumin, garlic powder, (cayenne pepper). Stir and cook on low heat for approximately 1-2 hours. Stir frequently. Add a touch of Mexican cheese and a few little pieces of avocado. *(I usually eat this by itself. If you'd like rice, limit it to no more than ½ cup of brown rice for the meal.)*

Shirataki Noodles

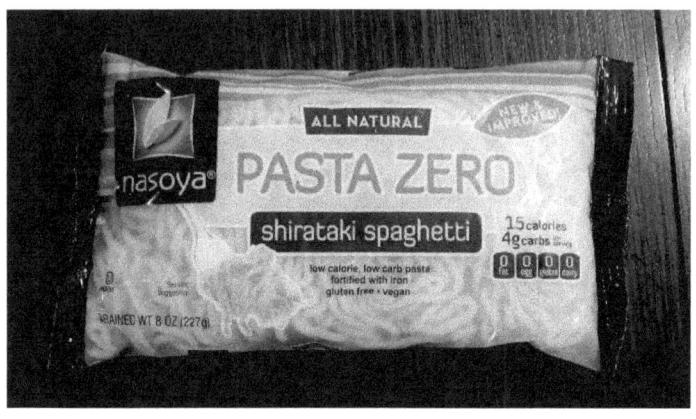

Have you ever heard of these? It's a great alternative to pasta! Shirataki noodles are a Japanese noodle – thin, chewy and translucent. Mostly composed of a dietary fiber called glucomannan, they contain very few calories and carbohydrates. They're packaged in liquid but have little flavor of their own, making them easy to prepare with many different dishes. Be sure to rinse them under cold water for about 5 minutes before cooking with them. Use them as substitute for pasta.

EASY DINNERS

Stuffed Peppers

4 bell peppers

1 small onion, finely chopped

1 glove garlic

93% lean ground beef *or* ground turkey

4 pieces of celery, finely chopped

¼ cup black olives

1 can crushed tomatoes

Italian seasonings

Garlic powder

Grated Parmesan cheese

Wash the peppers and cut off the tops. Scoop out the seeds. Spray a baking dish and set peppers inside. Heat a 3-qt. covered pan and sauté onion, garlic, olives and celery together. Set aside. Cook meat, until no longer pink. Drain meat and replace into pan with cooked veggies. Add crushed tomatoes and cook for another 5 minutes. Stuff the peppers and top with grated parmesan cheese. Bake at 350 degrees for approximately 15-20 minutes. Note: peppers will be crunchy. If you'd like them softer, microwave peppers in a covered dish for 5 minutes before stuffing

Healthy Eggplant Parmesan

I absolutely love Eggplant Parmesan. My mother makes it so good! But it's fried and not beneficial to your health. This version cuts out the frying step. And I'm proud to say that my mother came up with this healthier version. She has served it at parties and everyone loves it.

3 eggplant

Mozzarella (part skim), sliced

Ricotta (part skim)

Tomato Sauce (homemade, pre-prepared)

Olive oil cooking spray

Ground black pepper

Garlic powder

Oregano

Preheat oven to 400 degrees. Slice eggplant into medium-sized pieces. Spread on cookie sheets and spray with olive oil cooking spray. Cook until eggplant are soft to touch and tops are light brown. Let cool to room temperature. On half of the slices, place a dollop of ricotta, a slice of mozzarella, and a spoonful of tomato sauce. Use the other half of slices to cover the eggplant with the cheese and sauce. Once made into a "sandwich," add another slice of mozzarella and tomato sauce. Bake in the oven until the cheese melts.

Baked Barbecue Chicken

1 package of chicken thighs

Barbecue sauce*

Fresh ground black pepper

Garlic Powder

* This recipe is super easy to make but there's one thing that is difficult about it – finding a healthier bottled barbecue sauce. A couple of things to look for:

- No high fructose corn syrup
- No artificial colors

- Sodium around 300 milligrams
- 12 grams carbs or less per serving
- 10 grams or less sugar per serving

Put chicken thighs into a baking dish. Season chicken with pepper and garlic powder. Cover with foil and bake at 350 degrees for approximately 20-30 minutes. Spoon some barbecue sauce over each piece of chicken. Leave foil off. Bake for approximately 10 minutes more. Check to see that chicken is no longer pink. Serve with fresh vegetables and a salad.

Salsa Chicken

Another super easy chicken recipe. Great for a middle of the week meal when you're busy.

1 jar of salsa or fresh salsa (found in some supermarkets)
Chicken breasts
1 small can of olives
Chili powder
Fresh ground black pepper

Put chicken breasts into a baking dish. Season chicken with pepper and chili powder. Cover with foil and bake at 350 degrees for approximately 20-30 minutes. Pour salsa over each piece of chicken. Add olives on top. Leave foil off. Check to see that chicken is no longer pink. Serve with fresh vegetables and a salad.

Simple Grilled Chicken

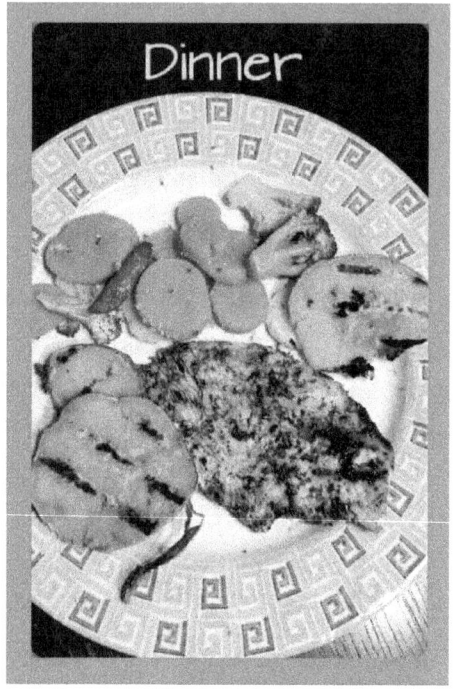

Grilled Chicken Dinner with Sweet Potatoes and Veggies

Whether you use an outdoor grill or an indoor one, grilled chicken is easy and healthy.

Grilled chicken

Fresh ground black pepper

Onion powder

Garlic powder

Preheat grill for medium-high heat. Season chicken with spices. Place on grill for about 10-15 minutes or until no longer pink and juices run clear. Serve with veggies and sweet potatoes.

Motivation is what gets you started.
Habit is what keeps you going.
- Jim Ryun

Chapter 7 - Motivation

Diet and exercise are essential for healthy living but there's another component – the mental aspect. Take your mind to a place of positives. Create your own personal power and motivation to succeed. You control you. You can't blame your husband for taking you out to dinner or your kids for not eating their meals and leaving you with leftovers. Temptation will always be there but you have a choice. Make a decision to be healthy and stick with it.

As parents, we tell our kids to always do their best. We tell them to put forth their best effort, and that "how you play the game" is more important than "winning the game." The same principle goes for adopting a healthy lifestyle. When women ask for workout and eating tips, I'm happy to share but they usually don't want to hear the answer. They'll say, "Oh, forget it. I can't do that." Or they say they're pretty healthy but they like to drink on the weekends, or they work out but eat whatever they want. Being healthy is an ongoing process with a series of ups and downs. It's not easy but, "nothing good in life is easy." Put in your best effort. Be willing to work for it.

Make a deal and stick with it

"How do you stay motivated? What keeps you going?" Everyone has different motivating factors. Find *your* motivation. In the beginning of adopting your new healthy lifestyle, it will be difficult. I tell you that because I don't want you to be surprised or get discouraged and give up. Life is hard. But it won't be the hardest thing you ever did in your life. If you've given birth, you know what I mean. That was hard. Or think about the millions of people battling disease every day. That is hard. This is difficult but not impossible. Being an adult is not always fun, but there are things we just have to do, like paying taxes, cleaning toilets, and going to funerals. You don't give up when you have an infant who needs to be fed every two hours even though you're exhausted. You just do it.

The first thing you need to do is tell yourself that this time you will stick with it no matter what the scale says or what happens in your life. Write it down on a piece of paper, make a vision board, record it on your phone -- whatever works for you. Make a deal with yourself. When things get tough, remember that deal. You are not going to give in to temptation and start over next week. Now is the time to do it -- no matter the day or month. You have to be strong and keep going. Stick with it and don't give up. You're doing it for you, so you can be healthy. And for your family, so they can have a happy, healthy mom, wife, sister, cousin, niece, aunt and friend. You are worth it. When you impose a rule with your kids, you can't back down. Treat this the same way. You can't back down from your healthy lifestyle plan.

After about two weeks, it will become a little easier. The hardest part is the beginning. You'll feel like eating as you adjust to your new healthy self. But once you are committed to a healthy lifestyle, it will feel natural. You won't feel the need to overeat and you'll be able to have a cookie, once in a while, for a treat. A taste, but not an over-indulgence. Embrace and enjoy being healthy!

Visualize your healthy self

You can stay motivated by utilizing a visualization technique. Visualize how you want to look and feel. Maybe it's an old picture of yourself from a few years ago. Perhaps it's a friend physique or a celebrity. Of course, if it's a celebrity, be mindful that most of those pictures are air brushed. Think about how you want to feel. Are you tired of being breathless walking up stairs? Do you want more energy? Are you bloated all the time? Wouldn't it be great to "feel" younger, vibrant and strong? Whatever it is, really see yourself looking and feeling a different way. Don't just think of yourself as overweight or out of shape. Begin to see yourself as a healthy person, whatever size that is for you.

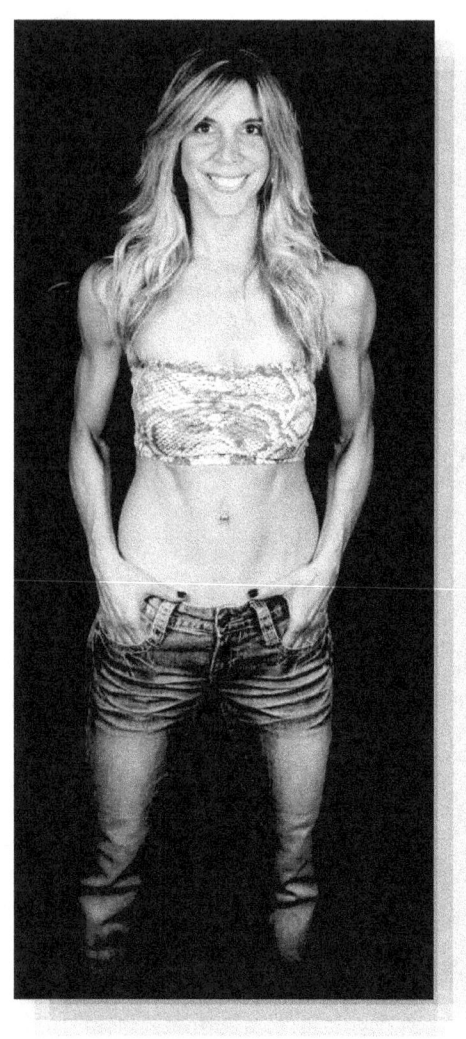

I use this picture for my motivation.
It was taken after I had accomplished my goal of getting healthy.
I remember what I was feeling: lighter, happy, strong, proud.
This picture has been criticized – too skinny, too muscular,
"too much." But it doesn't matter because I like it.
I like the emotions and memories it brings to the surface – fit at 40.

Thank you
Anthony Greco Photography

I always read fitness magazines and would see these beautiful, in-shape women. I didn't look quite like them but I wanted to have a similar look, one that fit my body type. One day I asked myself, "Why can't I look like them? What's stopping me?" The answer was, "Me." I was stopping myself. I knew I could change my body to look how I really wanted it to be. I had all the control and I visualized how I wanted my body to look. As I'm sure you know already, life can be difficult and there are many things that are out of your control: loss of job, death, natural disasters -- but you can control your body. You have to keep it as healthy as you can. Don't let "life" keep you down and don't find comfort in food.

Recently, I was talking to someone who had scheduled gastric bypass surgery. She told me she tried everything. She said she would diet for two weeks, then stop because she didn't lose any weight. Are you kidding me? Really? Only two weeks of "dieting" for years of eating badly and gaining weight. You have to give your body a chance to realize that you are serious. Many times you will not lose weight in the beginning because your body wants to hold on to that fat to which it has become accustomed. Sometimes you'll lose a couple of pounds of water weight, but you may not lose right away. Whatever the case, you have to keep going. Remember, this is a lifestyle change, not a diet with food restrictions. You are learning to become healthy, just as your children are learning algebra or how to play the piano. It takes practice and it takes time. Every day you continue to be healthy is practice for the rest of your life.

Surround yourself with healthy things

It's motivating to have people around that share your common interest. It can boost your confidence and inspire you to success. If you know people already into fitness, talk to them. I could talk about fitness all day and have found others that feel the same. Start to live the healthy life. Buy healthy, fresh foods like fruit, vegetables, chicken and fish. Visit a farmer's market for local produce. Read fitness magazines, borrow books from the library, read nutrition articles, peruse fitness blogs, watch exercise videos on YouTube, hang out at the park, try different gyms, and take new classes. It's a great way to get new ideas and get motivated. Sometimes we don't like new things because we don't understand them or have all the information about them. Understand why you are working out and eating healthy. Do whatever you can to surround yourself with all good things so it becomes a part of you, something that you are invested in, and something that's worth sticking to.

Make it a Game

Kids play games. As adults, we don't get much free time, but sometimes it's fun to sit back and just play. We've played solitaire, scrabble, angry birds, stupid zombies, trivia crack, and candy crush. They're fun and challenging so we keep coming back for more. Stay motivated by making it a game and by creating a challenge for yourself. You're in control and get to make all the rules -- but you need to stick to them. Each day, tell yourself that you will continue with this game and that you want to win. How do you win? You win when you don't give up. I'm sure you've taught your kids to never quit, right? Do the same! You can't quit because there are serious consequences to this game - your health and your life. This is your challenge. Don't be afraid of it, rather, embrace it and accomplish the goals you set. You will feel amazing after you've triumphed.

Establish a Routine

We all have routines in our lives. You wake up, give your kids breakfast, make the beds (sometimes), drive your kids to school, go to work, do homework, bring your kids to activities, cook dinner, bedtime. Something like that. Make fitness and eating healthy part of that routine. We manage our time and our family's schedules. You simply have to put working out on your calendar and make it part of your routine. You can't say you will fit it in if you're not busy -- because you'll always be busy. You can't say, you'll see how you feel the next day. You just have to do it. Somewhere in your life, there must be even a small amount of time to devote to working out. Don't use the weather as an excuse, or skip a workout because you had to work late. Tell yourself that working out is on your list and you need to fit it in just as you take time to eat your meals, drive your kids to school, check your e-mail and maybe get a pedicure. Even if you only have 30 minutes free, you can use those 30 minutes to work out. If you put working out on your schedule for Monday, Wednesday, Saturday and Sunday, then work out on those days. Yes, sometimes you may need to change your schedule, but make sure you switch your workout days, rather than delete them. Maybe try working out in the morning because no matter how busy you get, you'll already have your workout done. If you wake up 30 minutes earlier, you can squeeze in a workout and get on with your day. I know sometimes it's hard to get up early in the morning, but you'll never regret getting up early to work out. You'll feel much better after your workout and throughout the day. Once you begin getting up early to workout, your body will "listen" and you may find that you'll automatically get up at that time.

MOTIVATION TIPS

- MAKE A DEAL WITH YOURSELF AND ESTABLISH RULES.

- VISUALIZE HOW YOU WANT TO LOOK AND FEEL.

- SURROUND YOURSELF WITH HEALTHY THINGS.

- MAKE IT A GAME TO KEEP YOURSELF IN CHECK.

- ESTABLISH A ROUTINE.

Some people dream of great accomplishments,
while others stay awake and do them.
- Anonymous

Chapter 8 - Working out: It's not like gym class!

Do you remember when you were in school and you had to take gym class? A lot of people don't have fond memories. I remember having to wear a one-piece blue gym suit and it wasn't a good look for my short legs. I also hated getting sweaty in gym class and then having to put my clothes back on -- without showering. The worst was quickly re-doing my makeup and grabbing my Aqua Net to make sure my hair was still big and high (it was the eighties!)

Our Healthy Children

Thankfully, our children have a better experience now in gym class. Our kids are introduced to different kinds of activities that develop agility, endurance, strength, and motor skills. My son loves his gym class and looks forward to gym days, even when they run! I always ask him what they did and he loves to show me. I'm thrilled to see that his gym teachers are having them do burpees, mountain climbers, and planks. We should be doing these things with our children. We have the ability to show them a healthy way of life from a very young age -- a resource our parents didn't have. It was a different time and the information and opportunity wasn't readily available. Back then, it seemed like only athletes were physically fit.

Now, anyone, at any age, can be fit. That's one of the great things about fitness -- it's about doing, moving and action! As parents, we have to not only TELL our children, but we have to SHOW them how to lead a healthy lifestyle. It all starts at home and we need to set a good example for our children that includes moving and eating healthy.

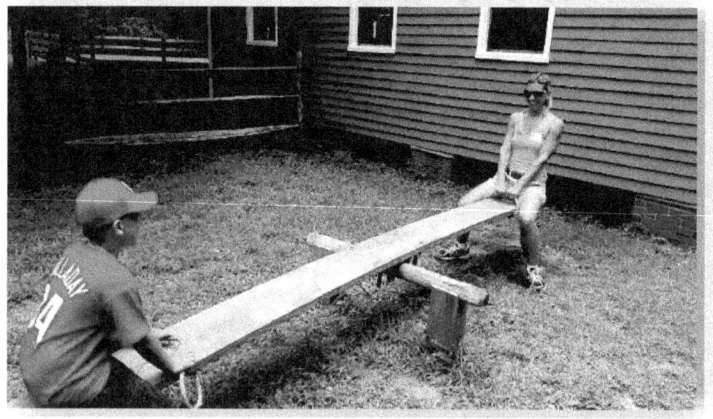

Playing with Jake – sometimes it's the simplest things

Here's some interesting facts about childhood obesity. **According to the Centers for Disease Control website:**

- The percentage of children aged 6–11 years in the United States who were obese increased from 7% in 1980 to nearly 18% in 2012. Similarly, the percentage of adolescents aged 12–19 years who were obese increased from 5% to nearly 21% over the same period.

- In 2012, more than one third of children and adolescents were overweight or obese.

- Children and adolescents who are obese are likely to be obese as adults and are therefore more at risk for adult health problems such as heart disease, type 2 diabetes, stroke, several types of cancer, and osteoarthritis. One study showed that children who became obese as early as age 2 were more likely to be obese as adults.

- Obesity is associated with increased risk for many types of cancer, including cancer of the breast, colon, endometrium, esophagus, kidney, pancreas, gall bladder, thyroid, ovary, cervix, and prostate, as well as multiple myeloma and Hodgkin's lymphoma.

That's scary and very sad. Since we know so much more now, why are children even more obese? Are they more sedentary because of video games, tablets, and iPhones? Is it because of safety issues where parents are concerned to let kids play outside alone? Are there too many "convenient" (processed, full of fat, chemicals, and sodium) foods that we are feeding our children? Are they not getting enough sleep because they are over scheduled? There are many factors and it varies from family to family.

I try every day to give my son the tools to live a healthy life. Some days work better than others. I know it's unrealistic to think he will never eat one of those sugary cupcakes. They look so good, right? But, I want to teach him to have just ONE, occasionally, even if an adult offers him another.

We are fortunate that we live close to my son's school so we walk as a family. It's about a 15 minute walk in one direction and he loves it. We started right from kindergarten. It's our family time (the dog is included) and we talk and make friends along the way, chatting with the school crossing guards and neighbors. I know sometimes it's not possible because of work schedules or the distance of the school but if you are fortunate enough to have this opportunity, take advantage of it.

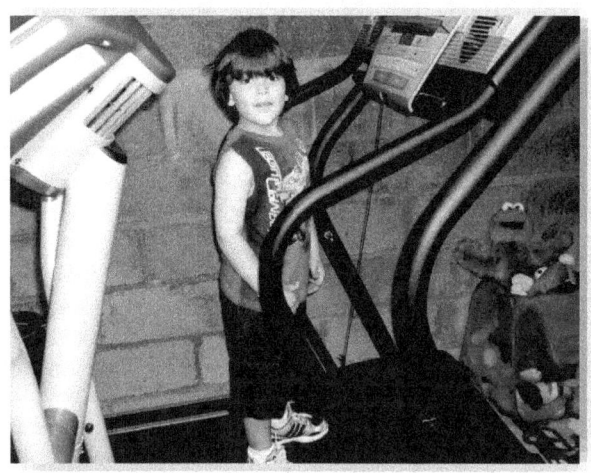

He wanted to be like mommy.

The Wonderful World of Working Out

There is not a one size fits all when it comes to working out. Everyone has their own goals, strengths and abilities. Some people like to do it and others don't. One person's advanced level is another person's beginner. And everyone has their own reason for working out.

When I first started writing this book, I wasn't officially teaching classes, but at the age of 41, I became a certified fitness instructor. I had always wanted to do it. The only thing stopping me, was me! At first, I wasn't sure if I could do it, if I should do it or how to do it. I realized that just because it seemed like a difficult task, it didn't give me an excuse not to try. I was writing a book to motivate women and I had to take my own advice. I was excited and nervous. I slowly researched the organizations and certifications, studied a lot and passed the practical and written exams. I teach several different types of classes and I absolutely love it. It's so rewarding to help others achieve their goals. The students in my classes are so motivating to me. I'm in awe of their dedication on an early, cold Sunday morning, working hard throughout the entire workout. I'm fortunate to have my day job working in a special education high school and I tutor ESL students, while also living my fitness dream.

It would be wonderful if everyone enjoyed exercising, but that's not always the case. Often people will tell me that they hate working out. I always ask them why and many times, they really can't give me a definitive answer. They'll say, "I just don't like it." "I'm too tired to work out." or "It's boring." That last response was from my own mother. But those are not good answers. There aren't any good answers for not working out. There are many different types of workouts that everyone should be able to find something they enjoy. When people think of working out, often times they bring their own negative past experience into their thoughts. Those bad thoughts may go back to their old elementary gym school days, or to a time when they tried to work out but weren't well-enough informed so it was a frustrating experience. That's similar to anything in life.

Long ago when I was trying unsuccessfully to conceive, on a whim, my husband and I adopted a puppy. We thought it would cheer us up, but we didn't know anything about having a puppy. We didn't know how to properly train it, we didn't have any information on the actual dog and we didn't have any necessary essentials like a crate or a leash. On top of it, my husband was allergic to the dog. It was disastrous and we were ill-prepared for such a big responsibility. We ended up giving the puppy back after only two days and we were crushed. About five years later, we now had our son and he begged me for a dog. I didn't want one because I had such a bad experience the first time but my husband assured me this time would be different and it was. This time, we researched the type of dog, an American Hairless Terrier that is hypoallergenic and great for people with allergies and with kids. We read books, signed up for puppy classes and made a trip to the pet store to buy all the essentials. We were well-informed and it made the task of training the dog much easier. The result is Lola who is not only our dog, but my "baby girl" as I affectionately call her. She is well-trained, great with kids, friendly and loved by anyone who meets her. The whole "dog thing," which at first was a bad experience, turned into a great experience.

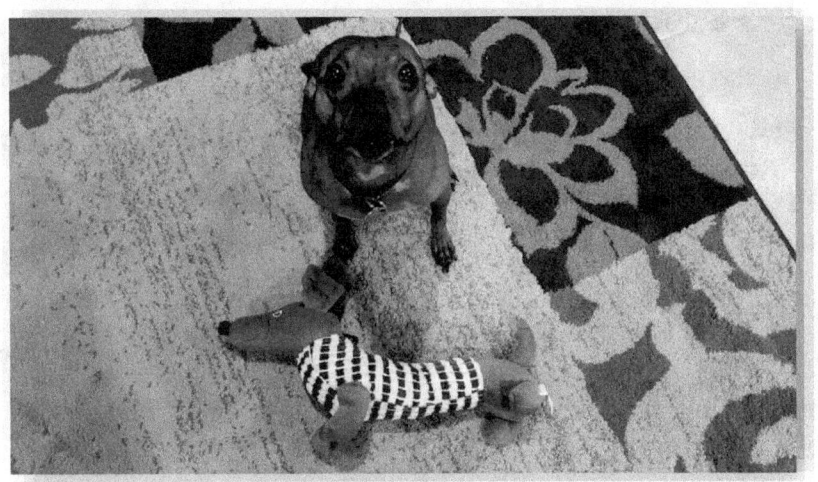

Lola poses for the camera

Working out could a great experience for you. Turn all of those negative, bad feelings you have about working out into a positive, wonderful experience.

Some women don't like to work out because they're out of shape. Even the thought of working out is daunting. Many times, when a person is unfit, working out is uncomfortable. Often, first-time exercisers give up because they feel terrible and never want to do it again. My advice: start out slowly with your workouts. Maybe the first week you only workout for 15 minutes. Do a few jumping jacks, take a walk, do some simple stretches, that's it. The next week, do a few more jumping jacks, take a longer walk, and maybe work out for 20 minutes. The week after, add in some squats and do one more jumping jack than you did the time before. You get the idea, right? If you were teaching your children how to swim, you wouldn't just throw them into the deep end. Instead, you would bring them into the shallow end, gradually moving to the other side. The same principle applies. If you are a first-time exerciser, start slowly and make realistic goals. Your first few workouts should be short and simple so you can get your body used to moving. Make it a positive experience and be happy that you are working out. Find an activity that you enjoy and one that you can grow with. Be consistent to build up endurance and get stronger. Soon, you'll be ready to try different exercises and work harder.

Don't be afraid to try different types of workouts. Find what is most effective for you. This book has workout plans, but I encourage you to try different kinds of workouts to see which fits you best. Some people like classes, some people enjoy riding a bike or running outside, others rather take a spin class at the gym. It's just a matter of preference. I will share with you what I do and what has worked for me. Use the *Mommy Muscles* plan but feel free to tweak it a little. Most importantly, stick with it and find something you enjoy. Remember, consistency is key. Stay on the plan and continue to work out. Don't give up because it was hard. Instead, use that as a challenge and work towards conquering your goals.

One time, I decided to try a new class that consisted of high-intensity, aerobic coordinated dance and strength moves. I was lifting weights and running, but this was something different from what I had been doing. My body wasn't conditioned for it. The workout was definitely tough, performing high intensity jumps and turns when I was used to slow, controlled weight lifting movements. But, I refused to stop and take a break. I toughed it out and finished the hour-long workout with sweat literally dripping down my entire body. About an hour later I developed a headache but didn't think anything of it. The next week, I went back to the class and found it equally as difficult if not more, because now my body knew what was going on. But I was determined and kept going. Again, I developed a headache and realized I was getting dehydrated. The third time I took the class, I got smart by drinking a lot more water. I didn't get the headache and I had more energy. The next week I looked forward to the class and started shouting out the motivational phrases as the other participants did. Each week got better and better even though it was still challenging and I was still sweating. I felt accomplished because I persisted and I conquered that workout and it felt awesome. You can have that same feeling! That's the great thing about fitness -- you can try something new and you can always keep learning and improving.

A Word About Soreness

It is very common for beginners to be sore after a workout. Or for anyone to be sore after doing a different type of workout – something your body is not used to. If you're a marathon runner and lift weights for the first time, you'll be sore. That soreness may last up to a week. To ease the discomfort, try soaking in an Epsom salt bath, get a massage, or use a foam roller. There are two types of muscle soreness. One occurs during the workout and subsides within a couple of hours. This is caused by lactic acid production. When you exercise, your muscles aren't getting enough oxygen, so lactic acid builds up. You can break down the lactic acid by slowly cooling down and then stretching, which realigns muscle fibers and speeds up the recovery process after a hard workout. The longer you cool down, the faster that lactic acid leaves the muscles. That's why cooling down is so important.

The second type of soreness comes a day or two after your workout, called Delayed Onset Muscle Soreness (DOMS.) DOMS is caused by tiny tears that occur to the muscles when working out. Your muscles need rest, so it's important to rotate your workouts. Don't repeat the same exercises and fatigue the same muscles on consecutive days.

There will be times when you'll be sore before a workout. Often, once your body is warmed up and you start moving, you'll be surprised to discover that the soreness will feel better. It gives your muscles a chance to loosen up, and may shorten the duration of soreness. DOMS isn't going to happen all the time and don't let it stop you from continuing your workouts. If your legs are sore, train your upper body the next time you work out. Or simply go for a walk. Walking is always a good way to get the body moving again. Consider it an active rest day. Of course, if you have a pulled muscle or have injured yourself, that's a different story. In those cases, you should not exercise.

Always check with your physician to make sure you are cleared for working out. As long as you feel good, try to make time for fitness. It can be an invigorating part of your life, helping you to feel energized, fulfilled and happy. There is nothing that feels better than having a good workout. It can make you feel good mentally and physically. You'll feel a sense of accomplishment, satisfaction and clarity. When you have a good workout, you should not only feel good about yourself, but you should feel proud. Pat yourself on the back, look in the mirror, and tell yourself that you did a good job. Each workout you do is a step toward being healthy and happy. Keep moving. Be consistent and find an activity you enjoy.

Working Out 101

I often get asked, "What is your exercise routine?" I have tried many different types of workouts and the one that I have found to be the most successful is weight training and HIIT (high intensity interval training). The combination of these two components has enabled me to stay lean and build muscle.

Weight Training

This is my favorite! Don't be afraid to lift heavy weights. If I had a dollar for every time a woman said they didn't want to lift heavy because they would get too big, I would be a billionaire. Women will not get big manly muscles because they are not genetically engineered that way. Women do not have the testosterone levels needed for major muscle gain. Men actually have 20 times more the amount of testosterone in their bodies than women do. Lifting heavy weights will get you nice, lean mommy muscles!

If you want to lose fat and change your body, lift weights. There are so many benefits to weight lifting.

- Helps raise your metabolism. Muscle burns more calories than fat so the more muscle you have, the more calories you will burn all day long.

- Protects your joints and builds stronger bones, putting you at less risk for osteoporosis.

- Increases your stamina so you can work out longer without fatigue

- Burns off an additional 25% of the calories you just worked during your weight lifting session.

- Can even improve coordination and balance and improve self-esteem. Plus, you'll see results pretty quickly. Sounds like a winning situation to me!

Basic Principles of Weight Training:

(1) **Warm up first for about 8-10 minutes**. Don't walk into the gym and just pick up weights. I see guys doing this all the time but you can seriously hurt yourself if your muscles aren't properly warmed up. A good warm up will improve your range of motion, activate muscle fibers, prep your muscles for work and increase your blood flow. You can do bodyweight exercises like jumping jacks, side lunges, squats and pushups to get your body warm. Then do the exercises you plan on doing with a lighter weight. For example, if you normally do bicep curls with 10 lbs. start off doing curls with 5 lbs. to activate that muscle. Often, I see people at the gym warming up using a treadmill or elliptical and then go lift weights. Although this will get your blood flowing, it is not a balanced warm up because there is no movement rehearsal or full range of motion movements. In other words, if you are lifting chest and back that day, you need to warm up those muscles too.

(2) **<u>Pick the right weight</u>**. Start with a light weight first. Work up to heavier. The weight should be heavy enough that you can only complete the desired number of reps (repetitions of that exercise at one consecutive time). The last rep, with good form, should be difficult. We'll talk more about reps later. For now, figure out the appropriate weight that will challenge but not hurt you. If you pick up a weight that is too heavy, you'll know right away as you won't be able to complete more than just a few reps. The norm is about 10 reps. Watch your form: don't use momentum, but rather use the muscle to control the weight. You need to feel comfortable with that weight, but it can't be too easy. Experiment with different weights in the beginning. You'll figure it out.

(3) **<u>Work the perfect weight</u>**. Once you've found "the perfect weight," similar to "the perfect black dress," I want you to work it, girl! You may be doing 8 reps and feeling good. Then you'll need to increase the reps to 10, then 12. Go as high as 14 reps. After that, increase the weight. If you start with 5 lbs. and can easily do 12 reps, move up to 8 lbs. and start with 8 reps. When working out with a specified amount of time, (E.g. 20 seconds), and those reps become easy throughout the work phase, then increase the weight. Don't stay with the same weight, because your muscles will plateau -- they'll adapt and stop growing. Please note: you'll use different weights for different muscle groups. If it's a leg exercise, you can go heavier. If it's upper body, use a lighter weight to start. And some days you may be stronger than others. Be aware of your body and adjust how you

feel.

(4) **Change the exercises that you do**. Just as you change your weights periodically, change the exercises you do. *Mommy Muscles* has different plans. Understand that you are not going to be doing the same exercises every workout. These plans will vary the exercises and the body parts you train together. Make each workout count towards reaching your goal.

(5) **Rest your muscles**. Resting the muscles is paramount in weight training. When you lift weights, you are actually making tiny little tears in the muscles. What makes the muscles grow and change is when they have an adequate rest. If you are lifting heavy and concentrating on specific muscle groups, for example, an entire session of biceps and back, then those muscles definitely will need rest. If your weights are lighter and you're doing it in an interval training format, it's okay to train on consecutive days. My workout plans will include different exercises so that the body doesn't have the same stress placed on the same tissues, in the same manner.

Reps and Sets:

"Reps" are short for "repetitions" -- one complete movement of an exercise. A "set" is the number of "reps" in a group. If you were doing bicep curls, one bicep curl would be a rep and you may be able to complete ten reps. Those ten reps would be a set of that exercise. You would rest and stretch for a few minutes before you start your next set, which may also be ten reps, possibly less if the muscle is fatigued. A goal would be to complete three sets of an exercise with ten reps each. Of course, that varies based on many factors, such as your fitness level, the weight you're using, and the other exercises you're doing in your workout.

By now, I hope I've at least piqued your interest in weight training. Learning is a first step to feeling more comfortable. Give it a try. It will only benefit your health -- and you'll be happy with the results if you stick with it.

HIIT (High Intensity Interval Training) and Interval Training

Interval Training is alternating bursts of high intense intervals mixed with lighter, recovery intervals. The heart rate becomes elevated during the high interval and recovers during the rest period. HIIT's method of intervals are high intensity with maximum effort in the high intensity phase. HIIT is all about the max. It involves alternating periods of short but intense exercise with less-intense recovery periods, therefore your body becomes a calorie burning machine. It's an exhilarating workout that you will both love and hate at the same time. The good news: you don't have to do it for a long time, sometimes twenty minutes is all you need. But the bad news: no matter what kind of shape you're in, it's a challenging workout. It's the new way of doing cardio. In a straight cardio workout, your heart rate stays within your target zone for an extended period of time. Your body adjusts to it. Whereas in HIIT, you're pushing yourself beyond the upper end of your cardio exercise zone so your body is working constantly. With HIIT, you increase your metabolic rate, causing you to burn more calories and that rate stays higher after your workout, resulting in continued fat burning. HIIT workouts are fast-paced and many times you'll use lighter weights or even just your bodyweight. You'll build muscle while increasing your anaerobic and aerobic energy systems.

Don't let the "high-intensity" part scare you. All movements can be modified. Remember - it's *your* max effort - not the instructor's or the person next to you. HIIT is effective and definitely powerful.

HIIT is the new way of doing cardio. What's the old way? Long cardio sessions on a treadmill or elliptical, staying at the same level the entire time - steady state cardio. Cardio training is based on the principle of longer term sustained exercise to build your endurance, your ability to continue, despite fatigue. One of the problems with this type of cardio training is that your body adapts quickly and the exercise becomes inefficient. If you continue doing cardio on a treadmill three times a week, you need to "change it up," either by increasing the intensity (adjusting the incline or speed) or, by varying the intensity, making it an interval workout. In the past, I used to separate my workouts into long, cardio sessions on the machines at the gym and then another day of weight training, never combining the two. I wasn't doing any HIIT training and I didn't get the results I desired. For me, a combination of HIIT and weights brought me to where I wanted to be.

Another problem with steady state cardio: misconceptions about how to fuel these long sessions. People often end up eating high-glycemic foods after it. They believe that because they walked on the treadmill for an hour, they can eat whatever they want. Often, they wonder why they haven't lost any weight. The reason: they haven't changed their eating habits and continue to do long cardio workouts. That "walk" was a comfortable steady pace - it didn't involve any change, therefore, the body isn't going to change. In addition, people feel comfortable jumping on the treadmill, hitting the same numbers, watching TV or reading a book. When it comes to working out, step out of your comfort zone. Otherwise, you'll always look exactly the same, because you're doing the same exercise, the same way, all the time.

Is long steady state cardio ever effective? Yes, if you're new to exercise. Doing 30-40 minutes on an elliptical or treadmill would help you burn fat. Once you are no longer a beginner, "change it up." I'm not saying never do long, cardio sessions. I am saying don't **only** do long cardio sessions. Change it up by varying the cardio, the intensity, and the time.

Tabata

Another term you may hear floating around: Tabata. A true Tabata workout consists of 20 seconds of high-intensity exercise,

168

followed by 10 seconds of rest, repeated continuously for 4 minutes with a total of 8 cycles. These are short but intense. If you don't have a lot of time, it's a great choice -- but in order for it to be effective, really push yourself to the maximum during the 20 seconds work phase. Tabata classes will offer a variety of exercises during a 45 minute or 1 hour class. Sometimes 2 different exercises will be a Tabata, other times it's 4 exercises or even just 1.

Circuit Training

You won't get bored with this workout. Circuit training consists of moving from one exercise to another, sometimes going to different stations and using a variety of equipment, for a specified amount of time. It's great for developing muscular strength and cardiovascular endurance. Similar to interval training in that, it can be completed in a short time. The exercises are performed one after another with little rest in between. This format is often used in the popular Boot Camp classes. You can do any type of exercises in the circuit.

Running

It's still popular and has been around for a long time. Just go outside on a sunny, spring morning or a crisp, fall evening and you'll see many people running outside. You don't have to run if you don't like to run. You can get into great shape with other workouts. If you have absolutely no interest in running, skip ahead. But, if you have a slight interest, or curiosity, and if it's something you'd like to get better at or something you'd like to try, keep reading.

Running is an example of steady state cardio, although you can absolutely turn it into a HIIT session. It completely depends on your goals. If your goal is to run a marathon, of course you need long training sessions. The only way to build cardio endurance for a race is by doing it.

For me, running was my albatross, something I always wanted to succeed at. I finally did but it was tough and challenging. What a difference it made in my body and in my mind. For as long as I could remember, I wasn't "good" at running and I accepted it, because it was hard for me. I hated cardio, especially running. I would say I had horrible endurance, and that's why I couldn't run. I would think I was trying but I never got past running a few minutes. As I got older, I realized that I needed to push myself beyond my comfort level to develop my endurance and change my body. I changed my attitude and I stopped putting limits on myself. Suddenly I *wanted* to run! I believed that if I wanted to be a true fitness enthusiast, I needed to be able to run. It was ridiculous that I couldn't and that I wasn't consistently working on it. I kept asking, "Why can't I?" I was the only person preventing that. It was a challenge that I accepted. I'm not a long distance runner and I'm not particularly fast, but I run. An average run for me is about 4-5 miles. Some days less, some more, with 7 miles being my longest. That distance works for my goals and it accomplishes what I wanted to achieve. You can do it too. Establish your goals and if you really want it, keep trying. Don't give up and don't settle because you are worth it.

Running isn't for everyone but, if it's something you've wanted to do and if you truly are ready to commit to it, then run! Start slowly. If you're on a treadmill, begin with a 5 or 5.5 so you can work on your breathing. As you progress, keep increasing the speed. Before you know it, you'll be averaging a 6.5 or 7.5! When you start, it will be difficult and you will feel like quitting, but you have to get yourself past that point. Your legs will hurt, your arms will hurt, and you'll be out of breath. But push through it and complete that run. Believe it or not, you'll feel great knowing what you accomplished.

Go for time. Try a walk/run routine where you walk for a specified amount of time, let's say 90 seconds, and then run for a minute. Continue the pattern for approximately 20-30 minutes. In the beginning, you'll walk more but as you get stronger, you'll run more. Set a goal. Run for 3 minutes and then take a break. As the 3 minutes becomes easier, start increasing your time. This is an effective way to increase your endurance.

Go for distance. Before your run, specify a distance you want to run. Maybe half a mile, a mile? Tell yourself that today you will run for that distance and you won't stop until you reach it. At an average pace, one mile is about ten minutes. Try to run at least as far

171

as you did the last time. Continue setting distance goals, gradually increasing your mileage.

Add intervals and hills. To make running into an interval workout, run at a faster pace for a specific time - 30 seconds, then recover for 30 seconds at a slower pace. If you're using a treadmill, you can program the intervals right on the machine. Running doesn't always have to be a steady pace. Change it up. Try running hills. Do it on actual hills or virtually on a treadmill. This adds a whole new challenge.

Positive Attitude. Running is not only physical but also mental. If you run and say, "Oh, this is so hard," you may have a horrible run. But if you have good music playing and a positive attitude, you'll have a good run. It can feel quite exhilarating. Get yourself into a comfortable, mental place on your run. Maybe it's thinking of a happy place or reliving a positive experience from your past. Let your mind settle in and exude positive thoughts. Some of my best runs have been at the beach or a local park. The setting is too beautiful not to enjoy the runs!

Machines at the Gym:

Weight Training - I don't use a lot of machines for weight training when I'm at the gym. Depending on the type of machine, they can be restrictive and only work one muscle group at a time. Most machines you "sit" and perform the exercise. It isolates the body.

172

There are times when I will occasionally use them but I'm all about the dumbbells. I'm a big believer in dumbbells. As a general rule, I prefer free weights (dumbbells, barbells) rather than machines. With free weights, you'll engage more muscles, especially the core. If you could only buy one piece of equipment, I would get the dumbbells. If you belong to a gym, then you have access to a plethora of equipment, some you may never use. If you have access to other equipment such as bands or a barbell, you can also use them to change up your workout. If you don't belong to a gym, it's okay. You don't need a lot of expensive equipment to get in shape. You can get a great workout with a minimal amount of inexpensive equipment.

Cardio – If you walk into any gym, you'll see tons of people doing cardio on the machines. Machines are fine to use as a supplement to your gym workout. It's okay to use them but don't *only* use them. Some machines can be used for your cardio workout and you can easily do an interval training workout with them.

Experiment and try the different machines to do cardio intervals. I want the gym to be a comfortable experience for you. Here's information on the basic machines you'll see in most gyms.

Treadmill: If you use a treadmill, promise me one thing... that you will not hold on! It's one of my pet peeves and it's cheating. It can cause injuries and result in unnatural movements. I constantly see people walking on the treadmill at the gym, holding on. This is wrong. It's not a natural movement. The exercise machines at the gym are designed to simulate the actual movement that you would be doing outside, like walking, climbing a mountain, riding a bike, etc. If you go outside for a walk, you can't hold on. Don't do it inside. When walking on the treadmill, you build your cardio endurance but, also work your legs and core by having good posture. If you hold on, you take that away. You'll use your arms to pull yourself through your steps and your legs and core won't be working. The whole session would be a waste of time. Remember, just like your kids do on their bikes, "Look ma, no hands!" Do the same!

StairMaster: Most gyms have some type of StairMaster machine that simulates climbing stairs. It looks like a revolving staircase. If I'm not running, then my second choice for cardio intervals is the StairMaster. It's an incredible workout and you can achieve results in a relatively short amount of time. The speed of the steps can be controlled. The slower they move, the easier it is, the more quickly the stairs move, wow - it's tough. If you try this machine and you're a beginner, start at a slow setting for just five minutes. Believe me, you'll be sweating. I prefer not to hold on because I like to walk upright to ensure that I'm working my lower body and using my core to help me move up the stairs. However, hold on if you need the balance, but don't bend over the machine. I've seen people hold on literally bent over the machine. That's not good form; bad for your back and not performing the exercise correctly. Just lightly hold the handles but remain in an upright position. Try to be as natural as possible. If you find yourself holding on too tightly, then it means you are fatigued and you should adjust the speed. Be aware of the position of your body and your grip.

Elliptical: The elliptical is easy on your joints and is a good machine for beginners. It has an upper body component - moving handles. Either hold the handles, moving your arms back and forth, or let go and move your arms naturally. All elliptical machines have a resistance setting. For example, a 1 is very easy and a 25 (the highest setting on my gym's elliptical) is the most difficult. Find the number where you can still move the pedals, but also challenges you. Let's say you can easily do a 4. Use the 4 setting as a five minute warm-up then increase the resistance to a 5 or 6 as you get into your workout. If you try a 7 or even an 8, and that's tough, do it for 30 seconds. Then go back to your 5 or 6. Use that number as a gauge and keep increasing that resistance number as you continue to work out. It's a good way to build up your strength and endurance. Too many people make the mistake of getting on an elliptical, punching in their usual number and staying at the same intensity for the entire workout. Their bodies are so used to that setting that they aren't even breaking a sweat anymore. It should be difficult and you should be sweating. Push yourself, but do it safely. You know your body best. When I saw that the maximum setting at my gym was a 25, I knew I had to get to that. The first time I tried it, I couldn't even move the pedals. I went back down to a 20 setting but I kept trying. Gradually, I worked my way up to the 25. Remember, when the resistance is high, you move slower, when the resistance is low, you move faster. Switch between low and high intensity to make it an interval training workout.

Stationary Bike: Another machine that can be used for interval training is a stationary bike. Most gyms will have two types of bikes, recumbent and upright. The recumbent is the one where the seat is behind the pedals as opposed to the uprights where the seat is above the pedals. Recumbents may feel a bit more comfortable but uprights give you the ability to lift your body off the seat and more closely resembles a bike you would ride outside. Try them and see what you like. Personally, I prefer the upright bike because it's the one most like a regular road bike and it best simulates an actual riding experience, Whatever you choose, really work it! I often see people on the recumbent bikes reading a book. Save the reading for after the gym, don't do it there. If you can read a book or check your e-mail on your phone, you're not working hard enough. Don't get "too" comfortable. Stationary bikes also have resistance settings. Adjust your intensity level so that you are challenged, switching between low and high intensity.

Spin Bikes: These are usually found in a group exercise class although some gyms may have a few on the floor. These bikes allow you to easily change intensity by changing resistance, pedal speed and body position. You can sit on the seat, stand on the bike or hover over the seat.

Personal Trainers

Most gyms will offer free personal training sessions when you sign up -- take advantage of it. The trainer will show you different exercises and how to work the equipment. If you can afford a personal trainer, that's a bonus for you but it's not a necessity to hire one. If you do, find one that is the right fit for your goals. Do research by checking out the types of workouts they use with their clients, read their bio and ask for testimonials. If you can, "watch" them with other clients because I've seen some uninspiring trainers. One of them was just sitting on a chair and drinking coffee while he was telling his client what exercises to do. Another simply stood there and counted the reps for her client in between checking her cell phone. A good trainer should be right there with their clients, motivating and pushing them to their fullest potential. The workouts should be fun and customized for you based on your goals and interests.

When you work with a trainer, it's easy to be "gung ho" while you're with them. But what happens when the sessions are over? I've known people who hire a trainer, use their sessions, and then never return to the gym. The trainer can motivate you -- but you have to motivate yourself too. Hopefully, this book will help you and keep you motivated. Think of it as your own personal trainer where the sessions never run out.

Also be sure that you fully understand the workout program from the trainer. Just today, I saw a woman attempting tricep kickbacks. She was doing them entirely wrong. Not only was her form off, but she was using a weight that was absolutely too heavy for her. I stood there doing my tricep extensions, contemplating if I should offer advice. I always hesitate because I don't want to make someone feel uncomfortable -- but I also don't want anyone to get hurt. As I cautiously walked over, I asked if she wanted some help. She said yes so I asked if she was doing tricep kickbacks. She said, "I don't know. I worked with a trainer a few times but I'm not really sure what I'm doing."

Ah! Even though she worked with a trainer, either there weren't enough sessions to give her a true understanding of the exercises, or she didn't have a good trainer. Something got lost and she was struggling. She won't get the results she wants, then she'll most likely give up. Be sure you fully understand what you're doing while you have the trainer. Ask lots of questions and take notes.

Breaking it down. Think of working out in 4 Steps.

Step 1 Warm Up - Always warm up before you begin exercising for approximately ten minutes. Start to move by using full body movements to slowly get your heart rate up and your muscles primed. Don't stretch yet and don't go full force. Go easy with the warm-up exercises, making them bigger as you feel warm.

SOME WARM UP ACTIVITIES INCLUDE:

- JUMPING JACKS
- BODYWEIGHT EXERCISES - SQUATS, SIDE LUNGES, FRONT LUNGES
- SHOULDER ROLLS
- DANCING
- WALKING
- LIGHT JOG
- JUMPING ROPE
- ELLIPTICAL
- BIKE
- STAIRMASTER
- PRACTICE THE LIFTING MOVES YOU'LL BE DOING IN THE WORKOUT WITHOUT ANY WEIGHTS

Step 2 - Go for it! - Do your workout and give it 100%. Get motivated, find your energy and have the best workout that you can. Don't read, text or chat too much. Focus on the activity and go for it!

Step 3 – Cool down - After the workout is complete, let your body gradually slow down, don't abruptly stop moving. Try "walking it out" in place so your heart rate gradually comes down. Re-do some of the warm up exercises without weights to cool down.

Step 4 – Stretch - Once your heart rate comes down a bit, enjoy a wonderful stretch while your body is still warm. It's important to stretch *after* your workout (not in the beginning).

Studies have shown that stretching reduces the risk of injury and soreness. It also reduces soreness felt the next day by decreasing the build-up of lactic acid in muscles. Often people don't stretch because they think it's not necessary, or they don't save time for it at the end of their workout. The obvious benefit to stretching is that it reduces muscle tension while increasing flexibility and range of motion. It also improves your coordination and balance by increasing blood flow to the muscles. This enhancement to your circulation helps to shorten the recovery time of injuries. In addition, stretching can aid in proper posture by keeping your muscles from getting tight. It can even act as stress relief by relaxing tight muscles that often develop from stress and increase energy levels.

Now that you know *why* you should stretch, let's talk about *how* to stretch. Only stretch when your body is warmed up or you could risk pulling a muscle, the exact opposite of what you're trying to do. When you perform a stretch after your workout, hold it for at least 30 seconds and be careful not to bounce. Bouncing can force a tear that leaves scar tissue, making the muscle tighter. You may want to time yourself in the beginning to get used to how long 30 seconds feels. It may seem long when you first start stretching, but after a while, it will be familiar and part of your exercise regimen.

The stretch should feel good; if it hurts, you've gone too far and you should pull back slightly. Don't force the stretch. As you get more flexible, you will eventually get further and deeper with your stretches. Be sure to breath as you gently stretch, never forcing the movement. Breathing is an essential part of stretching. It helps relax the muscles and aids in increasing the stretch. Inhale slowly through the nose and exhale through the mouth expanding the rib cage as you do so. Inhale right before the stretch and exhale as you perform the stretch. Pay careful attention that you don't hold your breath at any time during the stretch.

Your life will be no better than the plans you make and the action you take. You are the architect and builder of your own life, fortune, destiny.
- Alfred A. Montapert

Chapter 9 - The Workout Plans

Okay -- this is it... the actual workouts! All of these workouts have been tested by me and by a "test" group of women with varying ages and fitness levels. The study found that everyone enjoyed doing the workouts and they proved to be effective. Women were challenged but not overwhelmed. They felt the workouts were tough but "doable" and that everyone can benefit from these plans.

These workout plans can help you change your body. They have been created to utilize interval training performance with the most effective multi-functional exercises for strengthening and sculpting the whole body. These workouts consist of metabolic training (cardio fitness), muscular strength and endurance, core work, and flexibility training. You'll blast your muscles into shape by performing unique combinations and sequencing of a variety of different exercises using only dumbbells and your own bodyweight. These exercises can be performed anywhere at your own level to achieve maximum results.

After the listing of the workout plans, there are **detailed descriptions of each exercise**. In addition, you can view demonstrations of the exercises on my *Mommy Muscles* YouTube page - Mommy Muscles YouTube page. There are video playlists created for each workout plan. The playlist will run through each exercise in the plan so you can see it first. Then you can do the workout in the comfort of your home, adjusting the work and rest times for your individual needs to help you achieve your goals. Remember to keep challenging yourself. The workouts should never be easy -- that's why the word "work" is in workout. Keep pushing, ladies!

Fit in what you can, when you can. First, decide how many days a week you will work out. It's always important to make time to exercise, but sometimes it's just, "one of those weeks." Ideally, four days a week would work well. But maybe you have a crazy work schedule and three kids, so right now you can only workout three days. Hopefully, you'll be able to add more depending on the time you've allotted for exercise and your fitness level and goals. When you can, add another workout day in, even if you are only able to do it a few times. All of the plans are flexible and can be altered based on your specific goals and how busy your week is.

A helpful hint -- record your workouts. Keep a record of what you did for the day's workout. I write it down immediately after my workout, because I'll forget by the time I get home. Being a mother takes a lot of brain cells and sometimes the memory just isn't what it used to be. Something I've noticed more now that I'm in my forties. To make it easy for you, I've included a chart in the back of this book. You can use this to write it down, if you'd like. Record it on your computer, tablet, or phone, just be sure to capture the information. It's a great way see what you've accomplished and to chart your progress. One day, you'll say, "Wow, look how far I've come!"

Within each category, I have included 4 different workouts so you can switch it up. Mix and match the workouts as long as it's in the correct category. The workouts are divided into <u>Weight Training Intervals</u> and <u>Bodyweight Intervals</u>. In the <u>Weight Training</u> workouts, you'll use dumbbells for most exercises, except for the cardio bursts sandwiched in between the weight lifting. In the <u>Bodyweight</u> workouts, no equipment is required, but feel free to use dumbbells here too for an extra challenge. There's also a *Bonus Weight Lifting* section at the end of this chapter for those of you that want to get serious about lifting weights.

THE PLANS

Three-Day Workout Plans

Day 1: Weight Training Intervals

Day 2: Bodyweight Intervals

Day 3: Weight Training Intervals

Four-Day Workout Plans

Day 1: *Weight Training Intervals*

Day 2: *Bodyweight Intervals*

Day 3: *Weight Training Intervals*

Day 4: *Bodyweight Intervals*

Five-Day Workout Plans

Day 1: *Weight Training Intervals*

Day 2: *Bodyweight Intervals*

Day 3: *Weight Training Intervals*

Day 4: *Bodyweight Intervals*

Day 5: *Weight Training Intervals*

Six-Day Workout Plans

Do the Five-Day Workout Plan with the 6th day being an <u>Active Rest Fun Day</u>!

Go biking with your kids, take them to a park, play Frisbee!

The objective of the *Mommy Muscles* workouts is to utilize your time in the most efficient way that will challenge you and push you into working hard during the workout. They take into account your individual fitness levels and allow you to advance. These workouts use a method of timed reps, where you will do as many reps as you can during the prescribed times, then you'll have a rest time to recover. The goal is to increase your work time and decrease your rest time. Even though everyone will be doing the same workouts, they are customizable for you. This method will enable you to have a successful workout regardless of your fitness level and will always allow you to make progress.

To find your starting point, do each exercise (there are eight in each workout,) for 30 seconds, then rest for 30 seconds in between. If you're having a difficult time, increase your rest time to 40 seconds. You can go as high as one minute of rest. Make sure you have recovered enough so that you can correctly perform the exercises with intensity and proper form.

Similarly, if you don't feel that the 30/30 ratio is intense enough for you, decrease the rest time to 20 seconds, going as low as 10 seconds of rest. In addition, you can increase your work interval to 40 seconds, going as high as 1 minute intervals. (Note: you may find that during the weight training workouts, you'll need a longer time to recover. The bodyweight workouts will require a shorter rest time. It's okay to use different timing ratios for the different workouts.)

To progress your workouts, push harder during the work intervals. If you've been doing 8 pushups in 30 seconds, go for 10 or 12 during the same time period. Jump a little higher. Use heavier weight. Play with the time. Increase your work time and/or decrease your rest time. Keep track of your progress. (I've included a chart at the end of the book.) In order for the workouts to continue to be effective, you have to keep pushing and change things up. Experiment and find what works for you.

The length of the entire workout depends on your level. Aim to do each workout for 20 minutes to start, and up to 45 minutes as you progress. The work and rest times will change but you should always continue to cycle through the exercises to reach your overall workout time goal.

*You will need a mat and a timer
for both workouts.*

I suggest downloading a free app on your smartphone. Do a search for HIIT Timer or Interval Timer. These apps enable you to set up the intervals and even write the names of the exercises. The intervals can be scheduled and it will "beep" and countdown the time for you. If you don't have a smartphone, they sell interval timers you can clip on, or buy an inexpensive stopwatch.

Remember – warm up first and cool down with a stretch at the end. Set your timers – ready, set go!

Weight Training Intervals A - Dumbbells Required

1. Squats with Overhead Presses
2. Two Arm Bent Over Rows
3. Butt Kick Runs
4. Forward Lunges with Bicep Curls
5. Triceps Overhead Extensions - 2 Arms
6. Jump Front & Back
7. Reverse Lunges
8. Elbow Planks

Weight Training Intervals B - Dumbbells Required

1. Side Lunges with Lateral Raises
2. Chest Press
3. Mountain Climbers
4. Squats with Bicep Curls
5. Tricep Dips
6. Squat Jumps
7. Deadlifts - Bent Knees
8. Elbow Planks - Lifting Legs

Weight Training Intervals C- Dumbbells Required

1. Goblet Squats
2. Renegade Rows (modification on knees)
3. Squat Thrusts

4. Plié Squats with Bicep Curls
5. Tricep Diamond Pushups
6. Speed Skaters
7. Curtsy Lunges
8. Planks - Straight Arm

Weight Training Intervals D- Dumbbells Required

1. Walking Lunges
2. Front & Side Raises
3. One Legged Side Hops
4. Squats with Overhead Press
5. Triceps Overhead Extensions - 2 Arms
6. Scissor Jumps
7. Deadlifts - Bent Knees
8. Planks - Shoulder Taps

Bodyweight Intervals A - Dumbbells Optional

1. Jumping Jacks
2. Side Lunges
3. Mountain Climbers
4. Prisoner Squats
5. Speed Skaters
6. Planks with Body Twist
7. Jumps Side to Side
8. Plié Squats

Bodyweight Intervals B - Dumbbells Optional

1. Lunge Jumps
2. Cross Body Mountain Climbers
3. Curtsy Lunges
4. Squats with Front Kicks
5. One Legged Side Hops
6. Pushups
7. Bicycle Crunches
8. Jog in Place

Bodyweight Intervals C - Dumbbells Optional

1. Reverse Lunges
2. Pop Squats
3. Spiderman Climbs
4. Side Lunges
5. Jumping Jacks
6. Russian Twists
7. Mountain Climbers
8. Plié Squats

Bodyweight Intervals D - Dumbbells Optional

1. Squats with Side Leg Lifts
2. High Knees
3. Up/Down Planks

4. *Crunches - 2 counts up, 2 counts down*
5. *Burpees*
6. *Forward Lunges*
7. *Prisoner Squats*
8. *Scissor Jumps*

The Exercises

Below is a **Description of the Exercises** that are listed in the workout plans. Become familiar with them so you can move seamlessly through the workouts. Use my YouTube channel - Mommy Muscles YouTube page. to view demonstrations of each exercise. There are video playlists created for each workout plan. The playlist will run through each exercise in the plan. In addition, I've choreographed a warm up and cool down for your convenience. **Be sure to watch my quick video explanation of the Mommy Muscles workouts too!**

LEG EXERCISES

Squats - Stand with your feet a little wider than shoulder-width apart, your back flat. Bend your knees and hips to lower your body, almost as if you were going to sit in a chair. Keep your body up (don't arch forward) and heels on the floor. Move until your thighs are parallel to the floor and then push up through your heels to stand.

Prisoner Squats - Same as Squats, except place your hands behind your head.

Squats with Side Leg Lift - Same as Squats, but add a leg lift to the side. Repeat on both sides or alternate after each leg raise.

Squats with Front Kicks - Same as Squats, but squat, then add a right kick, squat, then add a left kick.

Goblet Squats - Same as Squats, but hold a heavy weight vertically in front of your chest. Keep your torso tight and aim to get your thighs parallel to the floor.

Plié Squats - Start with your feet slightly wider than hip-width apart, and your toes turned out about 45 degrees. Bend your knees and lower your body straight down, keeping your hips, shoulders and back straight. Your knees should be open but not past your toes, keeping your weight in your heels. Slowly straighten up back to start, keeping your core tight.

Curtsy Lunges - Stand with your feet hip-width apart. Take a big step diagonally back with your left leg, crossing it behind your right. Bend your knees and lower your hips (as if curtsying) until your right thigh is almost parallel to the floor. Keep your torso upright and your hips as square front as possible.

Lunges (Forward) - Keep your head up and your back straight. Step forward with one leg, leading with your heel and bend both legs, making sure your front knee doesn't go past your toes. Stop just short of your rear leg touching the ground but your front thigh should be parallel with the floor. Push yourself back up into the starting position.

Lunges (Reverse) - Keep your head up and your back straight. Step back with one leg and bend both knees to lower your body towards the floor. Your back thigh should be parallel to the floor. Push yourself back up into the starting position.

Lunges (Side) - Stand straight and take a wide step out to one side. Bend the knee of the leg you stepped out with until you are almost parallel to the floor. Your other leg, the standing leg remains straight. Push yourself back up into the starting position.

Walking Lunges - Begin standing with your feet shoulder-width apart. Step forward with one leg, lowering your hips toward the floor and bending both knees. The back knee should come close to the ground but never touch. Your front knee should be directly over the ankle not the toes. Switch to the other leg and move forward with the lunges.

Deadlifts - Stand shoulder-width apart holding two dumbbells (or a barbell) with your arms in front of you. Keep your knees slightly bent and with your back flat, slowly bend at the waist and lower the weights down to your shins. On the way back up, squeeze your glutes and return to the starting position.

CHEST EXERCISES

Chest Press - This exercise can be done on a bench, a step, or the floor. Lie on your back. Hold either a dumbbell in each hand or a barbell with both hands a little wider than shoulder width. Bring the weights to your chest, tighten your core and then lift the weight up. Do not lock your elbows. Return to the start position.

Chest Flys - This exercise can be done on a bench, a step, or the floor. Lie on your back. Hold the weights over your chest with palms facing each other. Keeping your elbows slightly bent, slowly lower your arms out to the sides, as if you were holding a big ball. Be careful not to lower the weights too low, stopping at chest level. Squeeze your chest to bring the arms back up to the starting position.

Pushups - Start in the "up" position (plank) with your hands slightly wider than shoulder-width apart. Tighten your core and lower your chest toward the floor in a controlled movement. Keep your back straight, head out (not down), and lower until your shoulders are level with your elbows. Lift yourself back up. If this is too difficult, start on your knees and work up to performing the exercise with your legs straight.

SHOULDER EXERCISES

Shoulder Overhead Press - Hold a pair of dumbbells to the sides of your shoulders. With palms facing forward, push the weights up until arms are extended overhead. Lower the weights back to the starting position. This exercise can be done standing or seated with dumbbells or a barbell.

Arnold Press - Hold a pair of dumbbells under your chin with your palms facing toward you. In one motion, press the weights up and rotate your elbows back, with palms facing out, as if doing a normal shoulder press. Lower the weights back to the starting position with palms facing in.

Front Shoulder Raises - Start in a standing position with dumbbells in each hand, palms facing your thighs. Keeping your core tight, with your elbow slightly bent, lift one arm until it is just about parallel to the floor. Slowly lower the dumbbell back to the starting position and then simultaneously lift the other arm. Continue to alternate lifting your arms in front of you. This can also be performed lifting both arms at the same time.

Side Lateral Raises - Start in a standing position with dumbbells in each hand in front of your thighs. Keeping your core controlled, lift the dumbbells out to the side with a slight bend in the elbow and your hands slightly tilted forward as if pouring water from a glass. Raise arms until elbows are shoulder height. Slowly lower back down to starting position. Make sure not to use momentum with this movement.

BACK EXERCISES

One-Arm Bent Over Rows - Use a flat bench or step and place your left bent leg on top of it. Or simply bend your front leg and support yourself on it. Hold a dumbbell in your right hand, letting it hang down. Pull it up on the one side, squeezing your back. Gently move the weight back down and continue your reps for that side, then switch to the other side.

Two-Arm Bent Over Rows - Hold a dumbbell in each hand with palms facing in. Bend your knees slightly and bend at the waist making sure your back is straight. Keep your head aligned. Lift the dumbbells to your side, keeping the elbows close to your body. Squeeze the back muscles at the top of the movement then slowly lower the weight to the starting position.

Renegade Rows - Hold a pair of dumbbells and get into a plank position with your hands on the weights and your feet hip-width apart. While pushing one weight into the floor, lift the other one into a row position, bending your elbow until it passes your torso. Lower the weight down and repeat on the other side. (Note: this is an advanced exercise so start with light weights or no weights at first. You can also start on your knees instead of your toes.)

BICEP EXERCISES

Bicep Curls (Facing Outward) - Stand straight with a dumbbell in each hand. Keep your elbows close to your body and rotate your arms so they are on the sides of your body. Lift the weights up to shoulder level, contracting the biceps. Slowly lower the weights back down to your sides. Weights can be lifted at the same time or alternate one at a time.

Bicep Hammer Curls - Stand straight with a dumbbell in each hand. Keep your elbows close to your body with your palms facing your body. Lift the weight up until your forearm is vertical with your thumb facing your shoulder, contracting the biceps. Slowly lower the weight back down to your sides. Weights can be lifted at the same time or alternate one at a time.

Bicep Front Curls - Stand straight while holding dumbbells (or a barbell), palms facing out. Curl the weights up to shoulder level, contracting the biceps. Control the movement going down. Weights can be lifted at the same time or alternate one at a time.

Cross Body Curls - Stand straight while holding dumbbells in each hand with palms facing in. Curl the right dumbbell up to your left shoulder, touching for a second. Slowly lower the dumbbell the same way then repeat with the other side.

TRICEP EXERCISES

Tricep Dips - Use a bench, step, a chair or just the floor for this exercise. Start with your hands slightly under the hips. Keep your shoulders down. Bend the elbows (the hips will follow - but be sure to lead with the triceps, not the hips) to about a 90-degree angle and then press down to straighten the elbows back to the starting position.

Tricep "Diamond" Push Ups - Start in the "up" position (plank), with your hands closer than shoulder-width apart, in a diamond position. Tighten your core and lower yourself toward the ground in a controlled movement. Keep your back straight, head out (not down), and lower until your shoulders are level with your elbows. Lift yourself back up. If this is too difficult, start on your knees and work up to performing this exercise with your legs straight.

Triceps Overhead Extensions – 1 Arm - Hold a dumbbell with one hand straight behind your head so that your arm is perpendicular to the floor. Your other hand can support by gently touching the opposite elbow. Keeping your elbow close to your ears, slowly lower the weight behind your head. Make sure only the forearm moves, the upper arm should remain stationary.

Triceps Overhead Extensions – 2 Arms - Hold one heavy dumbbell with both hands behind your head. The palms of your hands should be facing up. Keeping your elbows close to your ears, lower the weight behind your head. Make sure only the forearms move, the upper arms should remain stationary.

Tricep Kickbacks - Hold a dumbbell in each hand and bend over until your torso is at a 45-degree angle. Slightly bend your knees and keep your abs tight. Begin the movement by keeping your upper arms stationary, using your triceps to lift the weights until the arms are fully extended. Straighten your arms out behind you, squeezing the tricep muscles. Bend the arms back to the starting position. This can be done either one arm at a time or both at the same time.

CORE EXERCISES

Planks – Straight Arm - Start lying face down on a mat. Place your hands on the mat, arms straight, with your shoulders aligned directly over your hands, up on your toes. Keep your body straight with your head continuing a straight line between your shoulders and toes. Tighten your core - abs, buttocks and thighs and stay in the up "hold" position. The duration of the hold depends on your level. Aim for anywhere between 30 seconds to 1 minute or more.

Planks - Shoulder Taps - Start in Straight Arm Planks. Slowly lift your right hand and tap your left shoulder. Alternate sides. If this is too difficult, spread your feet a little wider for more support, or start on your knees.

Side Straight Arm Planks - Start lying on your right side with your legs straight. Extend your right arm, keeping it in line under the shoulder. Rest your left arm on your hip. Brace your abs and raise your hips until your body forms a straight line. Hold for 10 - 60 seconds. Repeat on the other side.

Plank with Body Twist - Start in a Straight Arm Plank and reach your right hand up, twisting your body into a Side Plank. Return to start position and repeat on the other side.

Elbow Planks - Start lying face down on a mat. Place your forearms on the mat (hands can be flat or clasped together), with your shoulders aligned directly over your elbows, up on your toes. Keep your body straight with your head continuing a straight line between your shoulders and toes. Tighten your core, abs, buttocks and thighs and stay in the "hold" position. The duration of the hold depends on your level. Aim for anywhere between 30 seconds to 1 minute, or more.

Elbow Planks Lifting Legs - Start in Elbow Planks then lift one leg at a time.

Up/Down Planks - Start in Elbow Planks, then alternate between Elbow Planks and Straight Arms Planks, moving one arm at a time in an up-up/down-down pattern.

Side Elbow Planks - Lie on your right side with your legs straight. Prop yourself up on your right forearm, making sure your elbow is under your shoulder. Rest your left arm on your hip. Brace your abs and raise your hips until your body forms a straight line. Hold for 10 - 60 seconds. Repeat on the other side.

Crunches - Start lying flat with your lower back pressed to the mat and knees up, feet on the floor. Place your hands loosely on the sides of your head, being careful not to pull on your neck. Lift your upper body in the crunch position, contracting your abs. Be sure to keep your elbows out and to control the movement slowly.

Bicycle Crunches - Start lying flat with your lower back pressed to the mat and knees up, feet on the floor. Place your hands loosely on the sides of your head, being careful not to pull on your neck. Lift your upper body in the crunch position and bring your right elbow and shoulder across your body while bringing your left knee in toward your right shoulder at the same time. Switch sides - left arm and right knee, making sure to contract the obliques - side abdominal muscles.

Russian Twists - Sit up straight on the floor with your hips and knees bent to a 90-degree level, holding a dumbbell sideways out in front of you. Either rest your feet on the floor or for a more advanced version, lift your feet off the floor. Twist your torso to the right, then to the left, with the dumbbell following, contracting your oblique (side) core muscles.

Spiderman Climbs - Start on the floor with your hands slightly wider than your shoulders and your fingers pointing forward. Keep your core engaged and bring your right foot toward your right hand. Return the right foot and then switch to the left side.

Metabolic Exercises

Burpees - Start standing with your feet shoulder-width apart. Lower your body into a squatting position, placing your hands on the floor in front of you. Jump both feet back into a plank position. Drop to a push up or hold in a straight arm plank for a second, then jump the feet back in towards the hands. Stand up and explosively jump into the air, reaching your arms straight overhead.

<u>Butt Kick Runs</u> - Run in place and kick your heels back toward your butt, one at a time. Swing your arms in a natural movement and be sure to retain good posture without leaning forward.

<u>High Knees</u> - Run in place bringing your knees up to your chest as high as you can, keeping your back straight, core right, arms moving freestyle.

<u>Jumping Jacks</u> - Start in a standing position, then jump to spread legs and raise arms high over your head. Return to start position and continue the jumping rhythm.

<u>Jog in Place</u> – Start in a standing position, then lift your foot and knee as high as possible to start the "jog." Swing your arms naturally.

<u>Jump Front & Back</u> - Jump with two feet front then immediately jump with both feet back. Land softly, knees slightly bent. Scoop your arms, using them to propel you to jump higher.

<u>Jump Side to Side</u> - Jump with two feet to the right side then immediately jump with both feet to the left. Land softly, knees slightly bent. Scoop your arms, using them to propel you to jump higher.

<u>Mountain Climbers</u> - Start on the floor with your hands slightly wider than your shoulders and your fingers pointing forward. Position one

leg forward bent under your body and extend the other leg back. Repeat and alternate leg positions in a continuous movement.

Cross Body Mountain Climbers - Start on the floor with your hands slightly wider than your shoulders and your fingers pointing forward but bring your leg across your body, reaching the knee to your elbow. Repeat and alternate leg positions in a continuous movement.

Squat Jumps - Start in a Squat and add an explosive jump up, engaging your core. Land gently, returning to the squat position.

Pop Squats - Start standing straight then jump into a low squat, sitting back into your heels, arms raised to shoulder level. Hold for a second then jump back to start position.

Lunge Jumps - Begin in a lunge position. Jump up and quickly switch leg positions in mid-air, while keeping your torso straight. Use your hands to propel you. Land in the lunge position, bending your knees to absorb the impact.

Scissor Jumps – Begin with one foot in front of the other. Jump up and quickly switch leg positions in mid-air, while keeping your torso straight. Use your hands to propel you. Land with your other foot forward, knees slightly bent. (This differs from Lunge Jumps because you start and finish with a slightly bent knee – not a full lunge position.)

Speed Skaters - Stand with feet hip-width apart. Hop to the right, landing on the right foot while sweeping your left foot diagonally behind your right leg. Swing your arms across the body. Switch to the other side.

One Legged Side Hops - Stand on your right leg and take a giant hop to the side, landing on your left leg. Your knees should be slightly bent and the hops should alternate quickly side to side.

There are literally thousands of exercises, all with different variations. I've included a variety of exercises to give you a good workout. As you get more comfortable, experiment with different variations. Change your exercises and tweak your routine. Remember -- this is your workout and it should make you feel good. Start slowly and do what you can. You don't want to hurt yourself and you should never feel sick during a workout. You may be tired and you'll definitely be sweaty and maybe a little sore. Push yourself but do it safely. Be smart and know your limits. You will get to know your body and trust your own instincts. When it gets really hard, just think how good you'll feel at the end of it. Keep moving. You can do it. I'm rooting for you!

Bonus Weight Lifting Section

If you've been working hard and wants to "shake things up," I've created special weight lifting workouts. You can add these into the routines you've already been doing with the interval workouts. Replace the Weight Training Interval workouts with these or add an extra day to your workout schedule. There are a few differences with these workouts:

(1) These workouts are straight weight lifting – no cardio moves and are meant to be done with heavy weights. If you use heavy enough weight and your rest is minimal between sets, you'll rev up your metabolism and definitely work up a sweat.

(2) This is not intervals, therefore, they're not timed. Here you will count reps. Start with 8 reps per set, working up to 10, then 12. If you can easily do 12, add more weight. In order for the training to be effective, the last few reps should be a struggle to complete.

(3) These workouts are split into muscle groups so you can intensely work and fatigue each muscle. The other workouts you've been doing are full body.

What's the same? You will cycle through the exercises in the same way – doing one and then moving on to the next, resting as long as you need but being mindful of keeping the rest as short as possible. Do the entire workout anywhere from 20 minutes to 45 minutes.

Weight Training Workouts- Dumbbells Necessary

Chest - Back - Glutes

1. Squats
2. Chest Presses
3. One Arm Row
4. Deadlifts
5. Chest Flys
6. Renegade Row

Legs- Shoulders - Core

1. Walking Lunges
2. Arnold Presses
3. Crunches (holding 1 dumbbell)
4. Forward Lunges
5. Side Lateral Raises
6. Russian Twists (holding 1 dumbbell)

Biceps - Triceps

1. Cross Body Curls
2. Tricep Overhead Extension - 1 Arm
3. Hammer Curls
4. Tricep Diamond Pushups

Chest - Shoulders - Triceps

1. Alternating Chest Presses
2. Chest Flys
3. Shoulder Presses
4. Front Raises
5. Tricep Overhead Extensions - 2 Arms
6. Tricep Kickbacks

Back - Biceps

1. Reverse Flys
2. Two Arm Rows
3. Bicep Front Curls
4. Alternating Bicep Curls (Facing Outward)

Legs - Glutes - Core

1. Goblet Squats
2. Plié Squats
3. Reverse Lunges
4. Side Lunges
5. Side Planks
6. Up/Down Planks

Time and health are two precious assets that we don't recognize and appreciate until they have been depleted.
- Denis Waitley

Chapter 10 - "Mom, I don't feel good."

How many times have you heard those words from your children, especially in the middle of the night? Getting sick is the worst. It's awful when it happens to your kids and when it happens to you. I know when my son gets sick, I feel like the world stops and my focus is entirely on him. As moms, we end up taking care of everyone, but it often seems that there is no one to take care of us when we get sick. I'm 40 years old and I still call my mom when I'm sick. Let's face it – we all get sick and sometimes need a little TLC!

According to The U.S. Centers for Disease Control and Prevention, more than 425 million cases of colds and flu occur annually in the United States. The average person has about three respiratory infections per year.

I live in New Jersey and winters are tough. It feels like every other day someone around me is getting sick and I am not immune. Unfortunately, when I get sick, I get "really sick" and it lingers. Often, I start to get better, go back to the gym, then get sick again, probably because I'm working out too soon and my body hasn't fully recovered. This is the wrong thing to do and I'm still learning from my mistakes.

I know people think I'm crazy but I get so cranky when I'm sick and can't workout. If it's for a long time, I start to feel "blah." Recently, I had bronchitis that started with a sinus infection and moved down to my chest. I felt awful, physically and mentally. Once I was feeling well enough to workout, my mood changed. The first time I put on my workout clothes after two weeks of not being able to workout at all, I literally looked at myself in the mirror and a big smile instantly formed on my face. I was comfortable and I felt like I was home again.

The big question is, "Should you work out when you're sick?"

The answer is, "It depends what you have."

If you have a regular cold and feel up to it, it's usually fine to do a reduced intensity workout. You could try walking instead of running, use lighter weights when weight lifting or do a shorter duration workout. However, wait a few days after the onset of symptoms. Don't work out the first couple of days, because the body absolutely needs rest. Colds often linger. If it's the 6th day, you might still have a runny nose, but you may be feeling strong enough to do a lighter workout.

If you have the flu, a stomach virus or a fever, that's a different story. Your temperature rises during workouts and if you are already running high with a fever, you won't be able to properly cool down and your body will be out of balance. Doctors say that if your symptoms are above the neck, it's generally okay to exercise and if it's below the neck, take a rest. Let your body be your guide. Listen to your body even if you don't like what it's saying! Be patient with resting and know that taking a break now, will help you become stronger in the long run.

On the other hand, don't rest for too long. Get back into it as soon as you feel well enough. Start slowly. Your body will be weak, but eventually you'll be back to your full strength. I've heard many women say they were in a good routine -- but they got sick and never got back into it. Before they knew it, six months had passed and they still hadn't worked out. Don't let excuses start creeping in. There are always going to be reasons. Being sick is one, but only for a short period of time.

While we are on the subject of being sick, let's talk about the "women sickness" as it was once called – your period and PMS. Ugh! It is so tough to be a woman and that's why we have to be tough. Once a month, we have to deal with getting our periods, PMS, bloating, cravings, and cramps. It is definitely not a fun time but you can still workout when you have your period. Usually the 1st and 2nd days are the worst, so maybe do a lighter workout or switch your workout days - don't stop entirely for a whole week. Even if you are not feeling 100%, do the best you can, alter your workout if you need to. Keep pushing and working hard.

PMS:

PMS (Premenstrual Syndrome) is defined as a group of symptoms, both physical and mental tied to a woman's menstrual cycle. They usually occur 1-2 weeks before menstruation. It affects women of any age and the degrees of severity vary greatly. Gynecologists estimate that approximately 85% of women suffer from PMS in some form. I define it as annoying and bothersome. If you go through it too, you know what I mean!

PMS Symptoms:

The physical can include a variety of symptoms such as headaches, bloating, soreness, fatigue, insomnia, and cravings. Mental symptoms can be anything from mood swings, irritability, depression, anxiety, trouble concentrating and memory loss. If you don't experience PMS, consider yourself lucky. If you do, adopting a healthy lifestyle can help to lessen these symptoms.

Eating healthy, will actually help your PMS symptoms. I know this is the time of the month where you may feel you need sugar or salt the most. But, if you are avoiding it the other weeks of the month, those cravings will lessen. If you really need that piece of chocolate, have a small piece. Don't let that one piece turn into a bag or box of chocolate, and definitely don't use PMS as an excuse to overeat. Make a deal with yourself that you will eat only one piece of chocolate and not another bite for the remainder of the day or week. You can also "mentally" plan ahead for the next craving by thinking of another food choice to have. How about sugar free pudding, a frozen banana or grapes, chocolate almond milk with protein powder -- just to name a few. Limiting sugar everyday will lessen those cravings. Make smart choices, be mindful of portions and minimize the damage.

Even if you're doing all the right things like eating healthy, working out and getting plenty of sleep, you may still be tired, bloated and suffer from headaches. Unfortunately, it's a bit of a battle for women. Don't be discouraged especially if you gain weight during this time. (I'll sometimes gain 3 lbs. but lose it as soon as my period is over.) It's not anything that you've done, it's your body going through the process. You can handle it. PMS is something we have to deal with but don't let PMS overtake you. Be in control, take a deep breath and stay focused on your goals.

PMS Tips:

- Eat smaller, more-frequent meals to reduce bloating and the sensation of fullness.

- Limit salt and salty foods to reduce bloating and fluid retention.

- Choose foods high in complex carbohydrates, such as fruits, vegetables and whole grains.

- Try to eat foods rich in calcium.

- Avoid caffeine and alcohol.

- Drink lots of water.

- Get extra sleep at night and/or take a nap.

- Exercise

Aches & Pains

We all get inevitable aches and pains, especially as we age. I call these "bumps" in my body. It could be problems with your back, hips, knees, ankles, or neck. Sometimes these "bumps" occur from working out. I hurt my foot while running, my shoulder from lifting, my thumb from bodyweight exercises and I've had my share of pulled muscles. When you exercise, sometimes injuries occur because we are human... not robots. This shouldn't deter you, but rather make you aware of "working around your injuries" and learning to adapt your workouts to be safer.

When I first started running, my right knee bothered me. It became so painful that I couldn't run for more than twenty minutes without intense knee pain, often hobbling home, and cringing every step of the way. One day, I mentioned it to my chiropractor, who had already been treating me with chronic lower back pain, and he said, "I can fix that." Each visit he would work on my knee and he was able to correct the misalignment. I remember he told me, "Now you can run as long as you want." And he was right. It's three years later and I'm still pain free.

I have some medical issues that I'd like to share with you as you may have similar problems. By sharing my experiences, I hope that in some way, I can help you. I don't have all the answers and I'm definitely not an expert. Of course, any information that I discuss here is strictly based on my own experiences and is not meant to provide medical advice. Though we may share the same issues, we are all unique in how our bodies respond. What I have are minor medical issues compared to what other people deal with. I know women who battle their bodies every day suffering from Multiple Sclerosis, Parkinson's disease, Type I Diabetes, Colitis and Scoliosis. But with their doctor's approval, they continue to work out so they can feel better physically and mentally. Try not to let limitations stop you entirely from working out. Rather, work around your issues.

Headaches: They slowly come on or appear quickly and painfully. Headaches can be triggered by stress, anxiety, sinuses, or lack of sleep or food. Regardless, they are annoying and painful. Depending on the type of headache you have, try to exercise. Many times, working out will help the headache. Sometimes I'll wake up with a knot in my neck and a pounding headache. As soon as I start moving and sweat, thankfully, the pain goes away. Of course, there are times when headaches become very severe, like a migraine. In this case, it's best to rest and speak with your doctor about your personal treatment. You know your body best. If it's just a little headache, try a workout and you may be surprised how much it can help. If it's severe, rest. When you feel better, resume your normal workouts.

Thyroid Disorders: The thyroid is a butterfly-shaped gland located in the neck that controls our metabolism. Its job is to secrete hormones which deliver energy to the cells in our body. When your thyroid does not function properly, it can affect every aspect of your health, including weight, energy levels and mental clarity.

The most common thyroid disorders are:

- Hyperthyroidism -- An overactive thyroid.

- Hypothyroidism -- An underactive thyroid.

- Hashimoto's Disease - An autoimmune disease where antibodies gradually target the thyroid and destroy its ability to produce thyroid hormone.

- Goiter -- An enlarged thyroid.

- Thyroid Nodules -- Lumps in the thyroid gland.

- Thyroid Cancer -- Malignant thyroid nodules or tissue.

- Thyroiditis -- Inflammation of the thyroid.

An estimated 20 million people have thyroid problems and sixty percent don't even know they have it. If you suspect you have a problem, see your doctor. It's a good idea to have an awareness of the issue and listen to your body. Sometimes you just don't feel right and if you're having symptoms, it's always a good idea to get tested. That said, I can't tell you how many times I have heard women say they hope they have a thyroid problem so their doctor can give them medication and then they'll lose the weight. Sorry, it doesn't happen that way. Although medication can make a difference, if you have a problem, you still have to eat healthy and workout. There is no getting around that and certainly no magic pills.

I have Hashimoto's Disease, hypothyroidism and a large nodule on my thyroid. I experience a lot of the "typical" symptoms, which include fatigue, infertility, irritable bowel, headaches, and muscle weakness. I deal with them and I don't let them change who I want to be. I do find that if I'm kind to my body by exercising and eating healthy, I feel better.

One year, I was extremely busy preparing for Christmas, decorating the finally finished renovation of my house, and planning a party. In addition, I was working, working out and volunteering at my son's school. I thought I could do it all. Once the "dust settled" literally and figuratively, I realized I was exhausted. If I was a celebrity, my agent would have booked me into one of those "rehab" places on the grounds of sheer exhaustion. To make matters worse, it was the holidays and I was eating some sugar. I felt like my thyroid was "out of whack." The nodule on my thyroid felt bigger and I was very uncomfortable. Shortly after, I got a sinus infection and a cold. I was a mess but I got better with rest. I didn't like laying around but my body craved it. I needed to treat my body right. I had been taking advantage of it and, unfortunately, I paid the price. The next year, around the holidays, I promised myself I would be better and that I couldn't do it all. Lesson learned. I was less stressed. My eating was right on target, only allowing a couple of days splurge. More importantly, I didn't get sick.

My thyroid is underactive and I take a loss dose medication to keep my levels normal. If you have thyroid problems, understand that it may take time to get it under control. Work with your doctor to get your levels into the normal range and then go ahead and change your body, your mind and your life. It can be frustrating but be persistent and be patient. Continue to work on adopting a healthier lifestyle which can help with the process. Don't use thyroid issues as an excuse to not workout or eat healthy. Rather, use it as a challenge, and be determined to overcome it.

Mitral Valve Prolapse: This is a heart problem where the valve that separates the upper and lower chambers of the left side of the heart does not close properly. The symptoms of mitral valve are palpitations, fatigue, shortness of breath, and dizziness. Approximately 10% of the population has some minor form of mitral valve and for most, it does not affect them. I was diagnosed with it in my thirties. I experience heart palpitations, a fast-beating heart and then a "flutter." The flutter is a strange feeling (similar to riding in a fast elevator that suddenly drops) that occurs when my valve get "stuck." I went on medication to control this, but it doesn't affect my workouts and I don't get palpitations while I'm working out. Most times, I can ignore it. I do notice that if I haven't gotten enough sleep, the palpitations are worse. I've learned that taking care of myself by eating right, working out and getting enough sleep, helps me. Keep that in mind -- it can help you too.

Stomach Issues: Irritable Bowel Syndrome (IBS) is a functional gastrointestinal (GI) disorder of the intestines with symptoms of chronic abdominal pain, fullness, gas, bloating with diarrhea and/or constipation caused by changes in how the GI tract works. Doesn't sound like much fun, does it? IBS is diagnosed when a person has had abdominal pain or discomfort at least three times a month for the last three months without any other disease or injury diagnosed. Basically, if you are having stomach problems and all of the tests come back normal, you are given a diagnosis of IBS. As long as I can remember, I've had stomach issues and I've been diagnosed with IBS. It's a fairly common diagnosis and some of you may have it too. Eating healthy definitely helps IBS though the types of food varies from person to person. Some can't eat broccoli and cauliflower. Others can't tolerate spicy or fried foods. I've found a few different foods that trigger my IBS and I try to stay away from them. If I eat them, it destroys my gut and takes my body a long time to get back to its normal, healthy state. If you find you're prone to bloating, eat smaller meals throughout the day. If the morning is a bad time for you, workout at night. It's a matter of finding out what works for you. It's not something you can forget about. It's always there, but work with your doctor and develop a treatment plan that is beneficial for you. Manage it by adopting a healthy lifestyle.

Insomnia: It is a sleep disorder that is characterized by difficulty falling asleep, staying asleep, waking up too early in the morning or feeling tired upon waking. From time to time, I suffer from insomnia. Through sharing my experiences, I discovered that many others do, too. It's an awful feeling and very frustrating to be tired yet not able to fall asleep. The worst is when you lay in bed, staring at the clock, and hoping to fall asleep for a few hours. Stress and hormones play a big part in insomnia. Learn to "close the door" on your thoughts to get a decent night sleep. Speak with your doctor regarding any necessary treatments. I've never taken sleeping pills but have taken a melatonin supplement if I am having a long stretch of insomnia. Melatonin is a hormone secreted by the pineal gland and plays a critical role in helping to regulate other hormones to maintain the body's circadian rhythms. Our bodies have an internal clock that controls our natural cycle of sleep. Melatonin levels begin to rise in the evening, remain high for most of the night and then drop in the morning. Sometimes our bodies produce melatonin either earlier or later in the day depending on the amount of light. In addition, natural melatonin levels drop with age and older adults may produce very small amounts of it. Taking a supplement can replace that lost melatonin and hopefully help you have a better night's sleep.

Insomnia can be frustrating, but continue working out. You may need to alter your workout but keep your routine. The physical aspect of it could help you with your sleep by giving you unexpected energy and also tiring you out. The mental component can make you feel better by giving you a sense of accomplishment and an emotional release. Who knows? It might actually turn out to be a really good workout. Blast your music and sweat!

We all experience medical issues, some more severe than others. Be thankful every day for what you have -- your health. You can't wait until you feel 100%, because that day may never come. All of us have problems and little aches and pains. Sometimes, there are serious medical problems that may hinder your goals. Always check with your physician before starting any program, especially if you have underlying medical problems. My philosophy is "stuff happens" beyond our control. We need to work hard on the things we *can* control. Once given the "okay," work hard to take care of your body. Eating the right foods can reduce inflammation in your body, give you necessary vitamins, minerals and other nutrients, provide you with strength and give you energy. A combination of good eating, working out, getting plenty of sleep and being positive is a winning combination for a healthy lifestyle. Be thankful and take advantage of your health. Treat your body right while you can. You are responsible for pushing yourself. Kick it into high gear - no excuses!

Just don't give up trying to do what you really want to do.
Where there is love and inspiration,
I don't think you can go wrong.
- Ella Fitzgerald

Chapter 11 - Be Inspired

Do you remember having to study in school? Did you have a teacher motivate you or have your parents push you to work hard? Do you propel your own kids to not give up, especially when they don't do well on a test? Do you do the same for you?

Now is the time to push yourself. That may mean something different for everyone. Maybe you want to be able to do pull-ups, lose the 30 pounds you gained with your children. Perhaps you want to get off your high blood pressure medication. Whatever "it" is, do it now. As moms, we often put our families first. As a result, we sometimes suffer. The best gift we can give to ourselves and to our families is to be healthy. It doesn't matter if your kids are babies or teenagers -- make time for yourself. Do you want to make a change? You deserve to feel comfortable and be happy with who you are, inside and out.

Be healthy and happy with your body.
Be the best "you."

We tend to put ourselves down for a laugh and have a hard time accepting a compliment because we don't want to seem conceited. Work on setting your goals. As you achieve them, set new ones! Keep telling yourself that you want to do better and you want to do more. Don't compare yourself to anyone else and don't feel like you have to compete with others. Don't stress about the woman next to you at the gym -- you're two completely different people with different body types, genetic backgrounds, and lifestyles. We are all at different stages in our transformations and in our lives. Women sometimes knock each other down to feel better about themselves. These women are insecure. Strong and confident women, who know their self-worth, lift others up. Once around Christmas, a group of women were talking about how badly they were eating and how they hadn't worked out in a while. I wasn't doing what they were doing so I just sat there quietly. Eventually, one woman said, "Oh, but not Jill, we know she's being really good." They all laughed. I replied with a simple, "Yes, but I'm a nut." I answered her question but also put myself down with those five simple words. I'm not a nut because I continue my healthy lifestyle around the holidays, yet I suddenly became vulnerable to the comments. I believe, these women, deep down wished they were eating healthy and working out. They didn't know how to do it or know where to find the motivation. It was another sign for me to write this book. There were times I'd get stuck and I thought about giving up. Family, work, and illness took priority. I needed a large chunk of time to write and that wasn't always available. Just like weight loss, this whole process was a long journey and lessons were learned along the way.

You are in control of your journey. Women say they are not

runners or that they'll always have fat legs or flabby stomachs. Sometimes they'll make fun of themselves. Stop! Don't label and limit yourself -- ever. Why do women do this? It's a shame that women can't just sit down and talk about how far they ran or what a great, healthy meal they made last night. Instead, it is more socially acceptable for women to talk about how they ate ice cream last night or haven't worked out in months. Learn to accept the compliment, then pay it forward. Recently, a woman who was in great shape, approached me at the gym and commented on my shoulders. She had nothing to gain and simply wanted to give a compliment. It was inspiring to talk with her about fitness. We shared tips and motivated each other. I actually told her she had a nice butt! I know that sounds strange, but from a fitness point of view, it's really not.

At my first gym, I made a great friend with a compliment. I had just joined and was working out with weights when I noticed a fit woman out of the corner of my eye. She was lifting a lot heavier than me. She was ripped and I admired her. I went and told her she had great arms and that I wanted my arms to be like hers. She thanked me and said she was a trainer and instructor at the gym, inviting me to her classes. I was nervous about trying the classes. Since she asked and was so nice, I decided to take her up on her offer. I tried spinning and boot camp classes and fell in love with them. I watched her in the gym, always helping people. I saw that she truly loved what she was doing. It was motivating being around her. We started working out together and I learned a great deal. She taught me different exercises and helped push me further in my fitness goals. I would also talk to her about my eating habits. During this time, I struggled finding that balance. She gave me great advice on healthy eating. She is a true motivator and we became friends. Perhaps this book can play that role for you. I'm trying to pay it forward. I want this book to be the friend that gives you advice and motivation to be the healthiest woman you can be.

My motivation now comes from helping other women. It truly makes me happy when women tell me I've helped them. I love hearing the stories -- it comes back full circle. When I first started teaching boot camp workouts with friends in the park, I had them run for three minutes. After a few classes, we doubled it. One of the women had never run before and was thrilled to discover that she was able to run six minutes without stopping. It motivated her enough to run on her own.

Another friend wanted to lose weight so I sent her motivational texts to help reach her goal. She told me those texts were reminders for her to stick to her plan. She enjoyed reading my inspirational and sometimes tough words. She said the one thing that really made an impact on her was when I told her that she was an intelligent woman, and that if she really wanted to lose weight, she could. I said she had already overcome obstacles in her life and it was time for her to work on her goal to be healthy.

A nice surprise came when a friend came to a fitness fundraiser

I organized at my son's school. She wasn't into working out but completed the class. Three months later she called and asked if she could stop by to show me something. I hadn't seen her since the workout. What she wanted to show me was – herself, 20 lbs. lighter! After the fundraiser, she told herself that if I could do it, she could do it too. Yes, exactly! She bought a series of DVD's and started working out in the morning. At first, she said it was difficult. But soon, she was hooked. She changed her eating and the weight just came off. In only 12 weeks, she lost 20 lbs. and went from a size 8/10 to a size 4. She had the determination and she is 100% into the healthy lifestyle.

Figure out what's holding you back so you can become healthy. If you're unhappy with your stomach rolls, your saddlebags, or your flabby arms, tell yourself that you want to do something about it. You can change all of those things with work. You can absolutely change your body -- but you have to put in the time and change your thinking.

When you start to get fit, other people will notice. They'll start to compliment you and you'll feel good about yourself. You'll have more energy, feel strong and be motivated to keep going. When you have a bad day, remember that good feeling. Create your own motivation. Working out is, of course, physical, but it's also mental. You have to get mentally into that place where you want to be.

Many women feel intimidated, scared and lost in trying to obtain a healthy lifestyle. Often, they bring childhood baggage with them into adulthood. Find confidence and be courageous enough to make a change in your life. Never be intimidated by anyone. There will always be someone richer, prettier, more muscular or smarter. That's life and that's okay.

I have a friend at the gym who's over 70. She looks like she's in her 50s. Not only is she in amazing shape, but she is the sweetest person. She has a positive outlook on life, she's always cheery and makes me smile when I see her. She is an inspiration. On the flip side, a twenty-year old girl at the gym told me she wanted a body like mine (the old forty-something year old). Don't compare but it's okay to be motivated or inspired by someone. It can make you work harder to get where you want to be.

Adopting a healthy lifestyle is a unique and personal experience. Maybe you're working out but haven't lost weight because you have bad eating habits. Maybe you eat healthy but have only been walking for your workouts. Or maybe you've been leading an unhealthy life in all facets and want to make a change. We are all at different points in our lives. It's your journey and life to live. Keep moving forward and you won't be wrong. Don't' give up. As you go through your personal transformation, you will have ups and down, good days and bad days. But it's yours and you own it. If you have a bad day, recover quickly. Don't let one bad day turn into three bad days. Celebrate the good days and reward yourself with non-food rewards. Your choice!

Some reward ideas:

- Mani/Pedi
- A good cup of coffee
- Watch a new movie
- Watch an old movie you love
- Read a good book or a fun magazine
- Look at old pictures of your family
- Play a game with your kids on Xbox
- Do a craft project with your family
- Call a friend (have a good old-fashioned chat fest)
- Peruse Facebook, Instagram, Twitter (without guilt)
- Listen to your favorite songs
- Watch those viral videos you heard about on YouTube
- Play with your pet
- Go shopping (one of my favorites!)

As cliché as it sounds, life really is a series of ups and downs, twists and turns, and surprises. All of us have gone through rough times -- life can be difficult. Why make it more difficult? Make it easier: Stay positive and lead the best healthy life you can lead.

Just as we continuously teach our children, we should be constant learners. Being an adult doesn't mean we should stop exploring with our minds, opening our hearts, and expanding our souls. Be open to new ideas and to expose yourselves to innovative teachings and experiences. Learn to love learning! Strive to better yourself and indulge in new experiences. Live life fully. It will keep you young. We've all heard, "Age is only a number." It's true. Keeping your mind young will keep your body young. Let's face it, we all want to be younger no matter how old we are. However, we have to appreciate the age we are at *now* because it won't last forever. Just look at how quickly your children have grown.

Recently, a friend asked why I was writing the book. She knew how much time I put into it. I told her I was doing it to help women to be healthy, strong, and happy. The past few years, I've spent my free time giving advice, planning menus, creating workout plans, teaching classes, motivating and listening. I knew I couldn't give up and the message is the same for you - don't give up ever! Be patient and persistent and you'll get results.

Homework

Every night we help our children with homework. Sometimes it's frustrating and other times it's rewarding. Nonetheless, it has to be done as it helps our children learn. Don't get nervous, I'm not going to tell you to do homework. But I will suggest it! A great thing to do -- keep a fitness journal or start a blog. Writing things down makes it real. It's a beneficial tool to record your workouts, daily food intake, thoughts and feelings. There are some wonderful phone/tablet apps that can help, like MyFitnessPal, MyPlate by Livestrong, Endomondo and JeFit. Search for food tracker and fitness apps -- many are free!

Food Tracker Apps: These help keep track of your daily food intake. They're great because they tell you how many calories you've eaten, along with important food breakdown information. You can even scan food labels. Just make sure you record ALL your food, not just meals. If you grab a cookie off the counter at work, remember to record it. It's a great way to keep yourself honest and to gauge exactly how much you're eating. Try it for a few weeks. The results may surprise you.

Fitness Apps: These give you a place to record your workouts. They also track how many calories you've burned and even offer workouts and demonstrations of different exercises. Newer on the market are activity trackers -- a device you wear that tracks your movement (both steps and miles), calories burned and sleep patterns. Some even have built in heart-rate monitors.

If you don't want to buy anything and you don't use apps, do it the old-fashioned way: record it on a chart or write it in a notebook. I've included helpful charts at the end of this book. Take a look or create your own.

Recently, I found a journal entry where I recorded how it felt to give up sugar. I wrote how tough it was the first couple of days and it brought me back to that time. It was just the information I needed to help a friend who was going to try it. We think we will remember, but we won't. Writing it down solves that problem and helps you see your progress.

Honors Class

Think of yourself in an Honors Class. To maintain that status, you have to continually keep challenging yourself. Push enough to achieve your goals but don't set unrealistic goals. That will only cause frustration and a possible "drop out." You can't jump from struggling to do a plank for 20 seconds, then the next time do it for one minute. Aim for gradual improvement. If you're new to running but want to enter a race, a marathon wouldn't be a good choice. Better would be a 5k, (3.3 miles). It's a natural progression. There may be a time when a full marathon is a realistic goal. You'll know when that is. Push yourself, but be realistic. It's not about doing advanced levels. It's about doing exercises correctly and getting benefits from each movement. It is not worth hurting yourself just because you're trying to be the best in the class or feel funny doing beginner moves. I'm happy when I see people in my classes doing modifications I offer. Everyone in class will not be doing the exact exercise. Everyone's at a different level.

Stand Proud

Pride: "a feeling or deep pleasure or satisfaction derived from one's own achievements, the achievements of those with whom one is closely associated." Often we show pride in our children's accomplishments and we praise them for a job well done. Children thrive from this acknowledgment. As adults, we should praise ourselves for a job well done. Be proud of the positive changes and the progress you've made. Don't focus on the slipups. Concentrate on the positive. Appreciate your body and be proud of who you are – inside and out. If you're unhappy with yourself, work to fix it, so you are happy. Don't make excuses. Take action. Set realistic goals and work hard to reach them. You may not love working out and eating clean but know you definitely will benefit from it. If you feel overwhelmed, make small changes. It will not be easy but it will be rewarding.

Know who you are. You may be a wife, mother, sister, caregiver and friend. Realize there are things you can change and things you cannot. Know your strengths and weaknesses. Every day work on achieving balance. My favorite quote is, "Work on your weaknesses until they become your strengths." So true! Many times we just accept our weakness but we don't work on them because it's difficult. It's easy to work on our strengths because they're things we're already good at. Working on our weaknesses is the real work. Try things that are hard. Keep challenging yourself to keep your body and mind strong.

External Traits: What's your physical appearance? Have long legs? Great skin? Shapely calves? What do you like about yourself? What can be changed and what can't be changed? I used to hate training biceps because mine weren't strong. Eventually I realized that I needed to train my biceps harder to make them stronger.

233

Internal Traits: How do you see yourself? Are you indecisive? Are you a gossiper? Do you have a temper? Are you shy? I'm not an adventurous person, but I wish I was. I'd love to go on amusement rides with my son but I can't. What I can do, though, is go on the bumper cars and have the best damn time looking silly when my car gets stuck. Appreciate and accept who you are while you work on improving.

Take some time and do a self-assessment. Do one before you begin your journey and after you've reached your goals. Compare the charts and see if you accomplished what you set out to do. I bet you did! Once you see that you have, you will be even more motivated to maintain your healthy lifestyle.

On the next pages, are two assessment charts for you: **External and Internal Traits**

EXTERNAL TRAITS

THINGS I LIKE ABOUT MY BODY	THINGS I DISLIKE ABOUT MY BODY	THINGS I CAN CHANGE ABOUT MY BODY	THINGS I CAN'T CHANGE ABOUT MY BODY

Internal Traits

Things I Like About Myself	Things I Dislike About Myself	Things I Can Change About Myself	Things I Can't Change About Myself

You have powers you never dreamed of. You can do things you never thought you could do. There are no limitations in what you can do except the limitations of your own mind.
- Darwin P. Kingsley

Chapter 12 - Good Things

Do at least one good thing for your body every day. Notice the "good things" around you. It's a great way to celebrate yourself and your health. Working out, of course qualifies as a good thing. So does eating fruit, vegetables and avoiding sugar. To lead a truly healthy life, surround yourself with positive energy and lead a life that you are happy with. Take care of your family and yourself. Over time, families change, kids grow up, our parents get older and we adapt. Do your best to be well rounded and healthy. Hard work is rewarded.

I am thankful every day that I have the health to do what I want and love to do. I realize that someday I may not be able to do everything. I don't have a crystal ball. What I do know -- I am doing everything I can now to make the future a better one for me and my family. Every day I focus on things I can control and pray for things I cannot control. I am grateful and humbled by all I've been given.

Little Details

As women, especially as mothers, we have to take care of the little details in life; buying birthday gifts, making sure toilet paper is in the house, washing kids' uniforms, and organizing the family

237

schedule. Take care of your own little details, too. Take notice of the "simple things" in life that will make you happy and make your healthy life easier.

Music: One of those little details that is important is music. There have been numerous studies that prove that music distracts you from pain and fatigue, while elevating your mood and increasing endurance. I always listen to music when I work out. Sometimes it's those same songs that you love, other times you may want to mix it up and listen to something new.

Music can change your mood and has the power to affect emotions. Lyrics can act as powerful affirmations and offer words of inspiration that can incite positive confirmation of your abilities. The right songs can give you the edge and help push you even further in your workout.

Take the time to find music that gets you motivated. Have fun, pick the songs that mean something to you, songs that will inspire you, move you and keep you going. Music can make working out a more positive experience.

Here's some all-time classic songs to help you get pumped!

Back in Black - AC/DC

Shook Me All Night Long – AC/DC

Eye of the Tiger - Survivor

Wild Side - Motley Crue

Kickstart My Heart – Motley Crue

(You Gotta) Fight For your right (to Party!) – Beastie Boys

Jump - Van Halen

Get This Party Started - Pink

Pump Up the Jam - Technotronic

Push It - Salt N Pepper

Gonna Make You Sweat - C & C Music Factory

The Cup of Life - Ricky Martin

Clothing: Whether you go to the gym or workout at home, you should feel comfortable. Of course, workout clothes usually are, but you have to be comfortable on the inside too. Wear something you feel "good" in, something that gives you confidence and makes you feel strong. Find your own workout style. Some people feel comfortable dressing in big, baggy sweatshirts, others like shorts and a t-shirt. It doesn't have to have a designer label or cost a lot of money. You are going to be moving around and sweating! Keep in mind that when you weight lift, it's a good idea to use a mirror. It helps to see the muscles you're working and to check posture and form. If you have baggy clothes on, that may be more difficult to see.

First thing in the morning, I put on my workout clothes. It puts me in the right mindset. These are clothes I only wear while working out, not to sleep, clean or go out to lunch. I think of it as a uniform. I feel like I'm ready to go and do my job. No backing down and no excuses.

Don't be too concerned with how you look. -- no makeup (maybe just lip balm), no jewelry. Hair pulled back or wear a hat or bandanna.

Sneakers (& Socks): This is an important little detail. You absolutely need a good pair of sneakers. In general, sneakers are expensive. If you're going to spend money, your feet would be the one place to do it. I know this from first-hand experience. Once I started teaching classes and doing a lot of jumping, my feet hurt. I got painful shin splints and it was very uncomfortable. I went to a running specialty store where they custom fit sneakers by putting you on a treadmill to analyze your gait, arch type, and foot mechanics. After the analysis, they suggest sneakers right for you. I also had insoles custom made and my pain went away. While I was at the runner's store, I tried a pair of nylon dry-fit socks and absolutely loved them. They have a nice cushion and keep my feet dry. They're only a little more money and definitely worth it.

Gym Bag: Another little detail to help make your life easier! Get a gym bag where you can keep your essential gym items. Sometimes I see women carrying pocketbooks in the gym and it looks strange to me. All gyms have locker rooms with lockers. Many gyms have locks built in or you can buy a small lock and use that to secure your personal belongings. If you don't belong to a gym, it's still a good idea to have a bag for your workout items. Everything will be in one place and it'll help you to get away from the distractions at home and get right to your workout.

Here's a peek into my gym bag:

Towel - To wipe sweat (Washed after every use.)

Almonds - In case I get hungry and need a little nibble.

Protein Bar - In case I'm very hungry and need more than a nibble.

Mints - Minty breath.

Brush, hair spray, barrettes, and hair bands - For getting hair out of my face.

<u>MP3 Player</u> - Gotta play that music!

<u>Deodorant</u> - Self-explanatory.

<u>Tampons</u> - Just in case.

<u>Body Glide Anti Chafing Stick</u> - Great product. I use it when I run, otherwise I get chafing under my arms. That really hurts.

<u>Weight Lifting Gloves</u> - I use them when I lift. If you are going to lift heavy weights, your hands will hurt and you'll develop ugly calluses. It's worth getting a pair.

These are the things that are important to my time at the gym. You may want different things with you. Depending what's going on in your life, you may add or take things out of your gym bag. When I first joined the gym, I carried diapers because there were times when the child care would call me over the loudspeaker to change a dirty diaper. I used to laugh and say to my guy friends, "I bet you never got called to do that at the gym." I was exhibiting my Mommy Muscles in the gym and on the changing table.

Graduation

If you have children, you might have gone through a few graduations with them. Kids graduate from pre-school, kindergarten, middle school, high school, and college. It's your graduation - you've finished reading this book. You have the knowledge, the determination and the will to make a change in your life. It's a new beginning. Your old life of being unhealthy and unhappy is gone. Your new life of being healthy and happy is here. I'm excited for you! You've invested the time to gather the information and taken the first step. The next step is up to you. You can start slowly by making small changes in your diet and exercise routines or you can jump right in and do it all at once. You are ready to be a new, healthier person. Work hard in the gym and the kitchen. Persistence and consistency are key. Strive for the best for you and your family. Be prepared to continually learn, change and grow. There will always be challenges -- do all you can to conquer them.

This book is written for you, my new friends. Use it as a reference, keep the workout plans section where you can easily access it. Re-read certain sections, as needed. I hope *Mommy Muscles* serves as a catalyst to change your life. I want it to motivate you to begin your own journey. I truly wish you the best of luck and hope you'll find the life you have always wanted and deserve. Let me know how you're doing. Please share your stories with me. I'd love to hear from you. Social media makes that easier now!

KEEP IN TOUCH!

Facebook: www.facebookcom/mommymuscles

YouTube: Mommy Muscles YouTube page.

Instagram: mommymuscles_jillthistle

Twitter: JIacobelli

When things get tough, remember your goals, hopes, dreams and family. You are a wonderful person. You can do this! All my best wishes. Be happy and healthy.

Family Pic

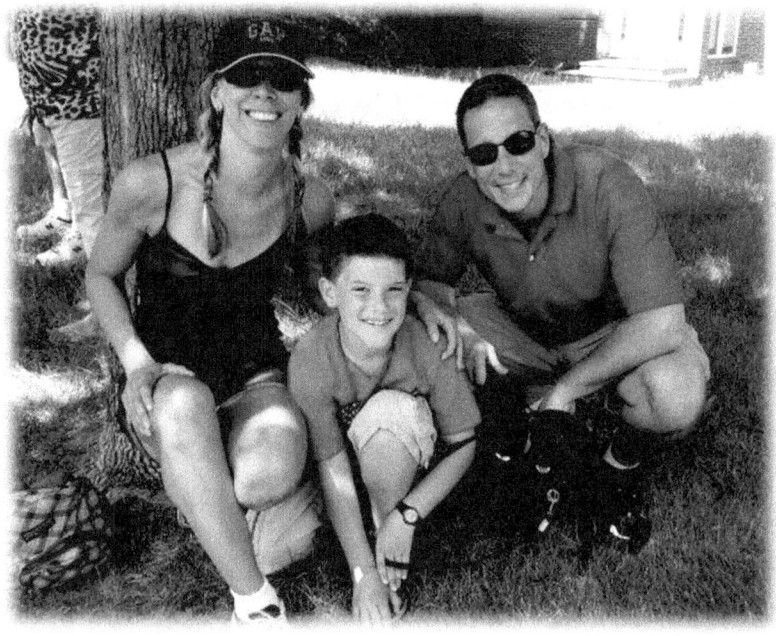

4th of July parade – all 4 of us!

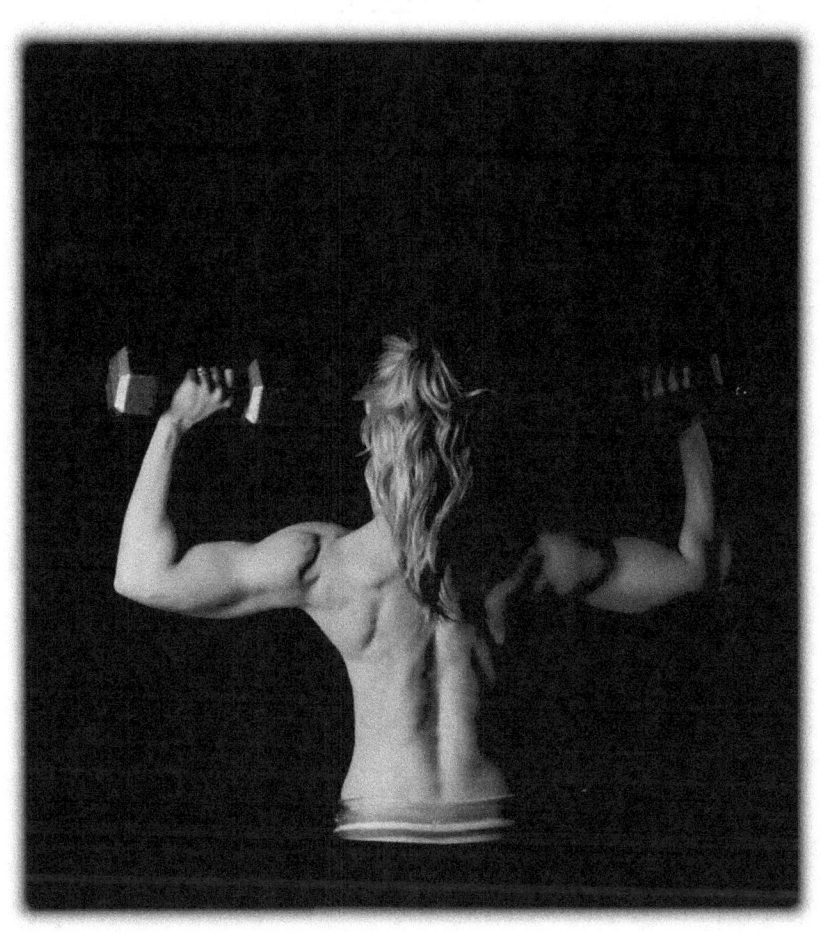

Anthony Greco Photography

FOOD JOURNAL

Week of: _____

	Breakfast	Lunch	Dinner	Snack	Snack
Monday					
Tuesday					
Wednesday					
Thursday					
Friday					
Saturday					
Sunday					

WORKOUT JOURNAL

Week of: _____

	Workout Plan	Weight Used	Work Time	Rest Time	Total Time	Comments
Monday						
Tuesday						
Wednesday						
Thursday						
Friday						
Saturday						
Sunday						

References

"A Low Carb Diet Meal Plan and Menu That Can Save Your Life." Authoritynutrition.com.

Berardi, Ph.D., John (January 22, 2014) "Eggs: Healthy or Not? Huffingtonpost.com.

"Childhood Obesity Facts." Centers for Disease Control and Prevention CDC.gov.

"Exercise Guides." Bodybuilding.com.

"Getting Healthy." American Heart Association. Heart.org.

Internicola, Dorene (February 11, 2013) "Exercise With A Cold: Is it Safe To Work Out While Sick?" Reuters.

Jabr, Ferris. (March 20, 2013) "Let's Get Physical: The Psychology of Effective Workout Music." Scientificamerican.com.

"My Plate." United States Department of Agriculture." Choosemyplate.gov.

Poliquin Group™ Editorial Staff (March 13, 2014) "Does Cardio Make You Fat?" Poliquingroup.com.

Quinn, Elizabeth (February 22, 2013) "Which is Better - Compound or Isolation Exercises?" About.com.

Roussell, PhD, Mike "Ask the Diet Doctor: Can You Drink Alcohol and Still Lose Weight?" Shape.com.

Shomon, Mary (August 26, 2013) "Thyroid Disease 101: Basic Information on Hypothyroidism, Hyperthyroidism, Nodules, Cancer." About.com.

Tallmadge, Katherine (August 30, 2013) "Eggs Don't Deserve Their Bad Reputation." <u>Livescience.com.</u>

Tallmadge, Katherine (August 30, 2013) "How to drink without gaining weight." <u>Health.com.</u>